CASTOR OIL BIBLE [10 IN 1]

Nature's Timeless Remedies to Revitalize Your Health Naturally. Soothe Aches, Strengthen Immunity, and Uncover Glowing Skin and Hair

LUNA MARIA SOLEDAD

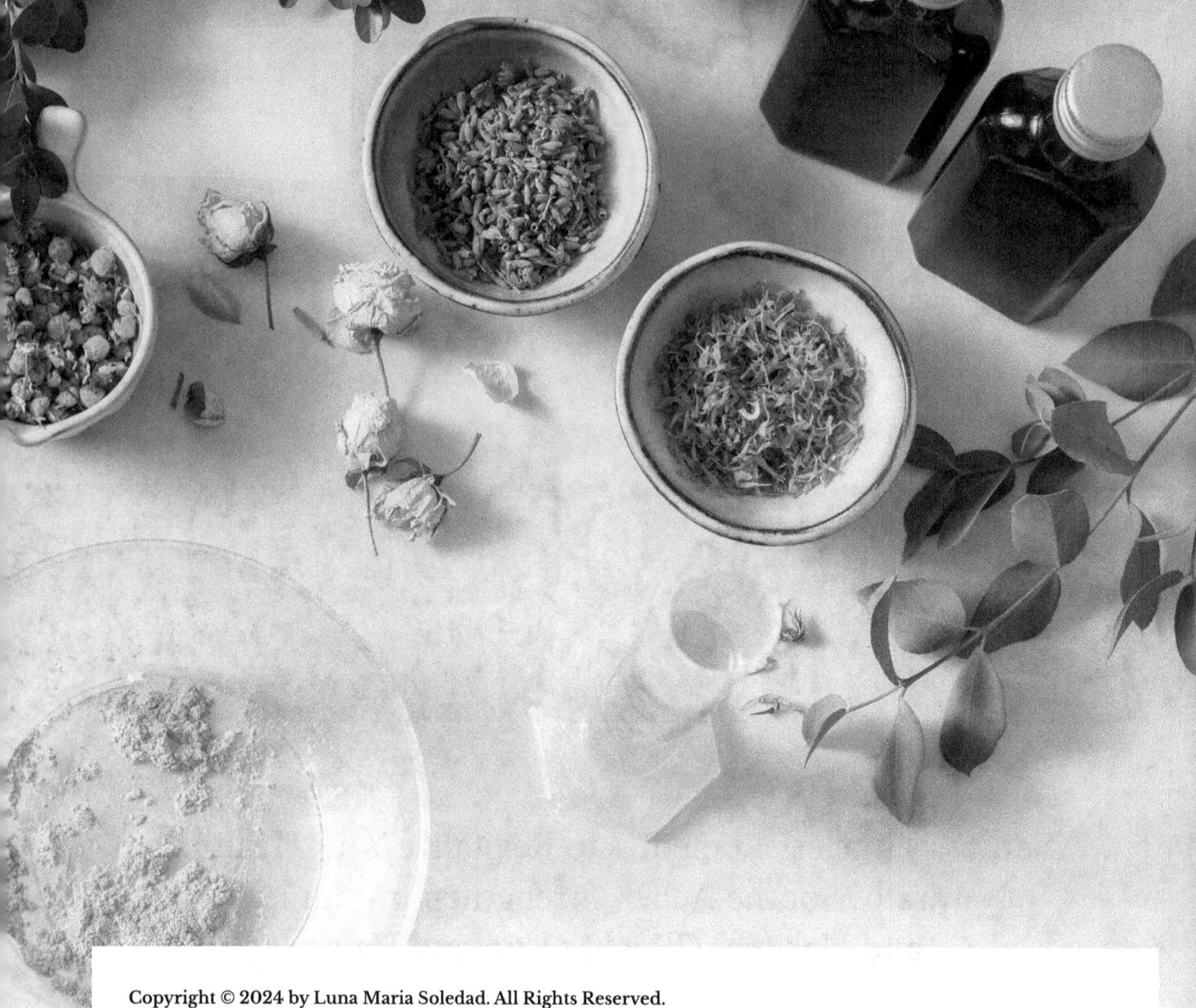

Copyright © 2024 by Luna Maria Soledad. All Rights Reserved.

This book, is intended solely for informational and educational purposes. No part of this publication may be reproduced, distributed, or transmitted in any form or by any means, including photocopying, recording, or other electronic or mechanical methods, without prior written permission from the publisher.

This publication is sold with the understanding that the author and publisher are not engaged in rendering medical, legal, or other professional services. If medical or other expert assistance is required, the services of a competent professional should be sought.

Disclaimer

The information contained within this book is not authored by Dr. Sebi himself but is inspired by his teachings and philosophy. This guide is a tribute to Dr. Sebi's legacy and is not an official publication from Dr. Sebi or his estate. It is intended to provide a practical resource for understanding and applying the principles associated with Dr. Sebi's approach, including the alkaline diet, herbal remedies, and detox protocols.

The author and publisher are not medical professionals. This book is not a substitute for professional medical advice, diagnosis, or treatment. Readers should consult their healthcare provider before undertaking any new health or diet program, especially if they have pre-existing health conditions, are pregnant or nursing, or are taking medication.

While the author and publisher have made every effort to ensure the accuracy of the information provided, individual results may vary. Neither the author nor the publisher shall be held liable or responsible for any errors, omissions, or outcomes related to the use of the information in this book. The reader assumes full responsibility for their own health and wellness decisions and releases the author and publisher from any liability resulting from the use or misuse of the information herein.

All trademarks and brands mentioned within this book are the property of their respective owners and are used for clarification and reference only. The author and publisher do not claim any affiliation with or endorsement by these trademark owners.

TABLE OF CONTENTS

INTRODUCTION 6
The Benefits and History of Castor Oil 6
Dr. Barbara's Holistic Approach to Health 7
Why Castor Oil for Health and Wellness? 7
Root Cause vs. Symptom Relief 8
How to Use This Book 8
Navigating the Book's Structure 9
Personalizing Remedies for Your Unique Needs 9

BOOK 1
THE HEALING POWER OF CASTOR OIL 11
Unique Properties of Castor Oil 12
Embracing Castor Oil's Unique Qualities 15
Scientific Benefits of Castor Oil 15
Embracing Castor Oil's Scientific Benefits 18
Remedies for Castor Oil Applications 18

BOOK 2
SKIN HEALTH AND ANTI-AGING 24
Daily Skin Care Routine 25
Anti-Aging Benefits 25
Remedies 26

BOOK 3
HAIR AND SCALP WELLNESS 32
Hair Growth and Nourishment 32
Scalp Treatments 33
Remedies 33

BOOK 4
PAIN RELIEF AND INFLAMMATION MANAGEMENT 39
Anti-Inflammatory Benefits 40
Castor Oil for Inflammation Relief 40
Pain Relief Applications 40
Remedies 41

BOOK 5
DETOX AND DIGESTIVE HEALTH 46
Digestive Support 47

Benefits of Castor Oil for Gut Health 47
Dr. Barbara's Detox Protocol 48
Using Castor Oil for Safe Detox 48
Remedies 49

BOOK 6
HORMONAL BALANCE AND WOMEN'S HEALTH 54
Hormone Balance 55
Supporting Hormonal Health with Castor Oil 55
Women's Health Applications 56
Menopause and Menstrual Pain 56
Remedies 56

BOOK 7
GENTLE CARE FOR CHILDREN 62
Safe Use for Children 63
Castor Oil for Common Ailments 63
Immune and Restful Sleep Support 63
Remedies 64

BOOK 8
MEN'S HEALTH AND GROOMING 69
Grooming and Skin Care 70
Castor Oil for Beard and Hair 70
Health Support for Men 70
Prostate and Muscle Health 71
Remedies 71

BOOK 9
ECO-FRIENDLY HOME AND CLEANING 77
Home Cleaning Solutions 78
Creating Non-Toxic Cleaners 78
Sustainable Household Products 78
Remedies 79

BOOK 10
PET CARE 84
Skin and Coat Care for Pets 85
Castor Oil for Pet Health 85
Natural First Aid for Pets 85
Remedies 85

APPENDIX 1
RELAXATION AND WELLNESS 91
Castor Oil for Relaxation 91
Stress Relief Applications 92
Self-Care Practices with Castor Oil 92

Remedies...92

APPENDIX 2
INSIGHTS FROM DR. BARBARA'S RESEARCH 98
Scientific Research on Castor Oil's Benefits 99
Real-Life Transformations with Castor Oil 99
Integrative Approaches 99
Remedies 100

APPENDIX 3
DIY – CRAFTING CASTOR OIL PREPARATIONS 104
Creating Herbal Tinctures and Infused Oils 104
Instructions and Tips for DIY Preparations 105
Personalized Castor Oil Products 105
Lotions, Serums, and Ointments 105
Remedies 106

APPENDIX 4
EMOTIONAL BALANCE AND MENTAL CLARITY 117
Techniques for Emotional Wellness 118
Castor Oil for Mental Clarity 119
Integrating Castor Oil into Your Emotional and Mental Wellness Routine 121

APPENDIX 5
CASTOR OIL IN SPORTS AND FITNESS RECOVERY 122
Benefits of Castor Oil for Active Lifestyles 123
Castor Oil for Muscle Recovery and Flexibility 124
Remedies for Sports and Fitness Recovery 125
Integrating Castor Oil into a Sports and Fitness Recovery Routine 127

CONCLUSION 128

YOUR EXCLUSIVE BONUS 131

INDEX 132

INTRODUCTION

Welcome to a journey into the world of castor oil, where nature's gifts align with our own deep-rooted need for healing and self-care. In these pages, you're invited to slow down and embrace the beauty of natural remedies—a world where powerful solutions often come from the simplest sources. Castor oil is one of those sources. Known and cherished for centuries, it has been a trusted companion for everything from nurturing skin and hair to soothing aches and supporting inner wellness. In a way, this book isn't just about castor oil; it's about reconnecting with ancient practices that honor the body's wisdom and resilience. As you explore each remedy, each thoughtful application, you'll discover how castor oil can be a steady, dependable ally in your life.

THE BENEFITS AND HISTORY OF CASTOR OIL

Imagine a time thousands of years ago, a time when ancient healers discovered that the seeds of the castor plant held something remarkable within them. These seeds, when pressed, released an oil that was immediately appreciated for its medicinal and therapeutic properties. In ancient Egypt, castor oil was revered not just as a beauty secret but as a healing balm used to soothe skin, improve digestion, and even relieve pain. Cleopatra herself is said to have used castor oil to brighten her eyes, giving them the iconic sparkle we still associate with her image today. This oil was treasured for its ability to restore and rejuvenate, to heal and to beautify—a testament to its versatility and potency.

Castor oil's story doesn't end in Egypt. Across the Indian subcontinent, Ayurvedic practitioners recognized castor oil's deeply purifying qualities. They saw it as a tool for cleansing, something that could restore balance within the body by easing digestive discomforts and relieving joint pain. In many ways, castor oil was viewed as a sacred remedy, a substance that could bring harmony to the body by addressing both physical and energetic imbalances. Its role in Ayurveda remains significant to this day, reflecting the oil's ability to transcend time and culture.

Fast forward to today, and castor oil has once again found its way into the hearts and homes of people seeking natural solutions. Scientific research has caught up with ancient wisdom, confirming what people have known for centuries: castor oil works. It is uniquely rich in ricinoleic acid, an omega-9 fatty acid that has powerful anti-inflammatory and antimicrobial properties. This makes castor oil exceptional at soothing skin, reducing inflammation, and even fighting bacteria.

Its vitamin E content supports cellular regeneration, making it ideal for wound healing and skincare. This oil is a gift from nature, one that offers benefits as relevant today as they were millennia ago.

DR. BARBARA'S HOLISTIC APPROACH TO HEALTH

To truly unlock the potential of castor oil, Dr. Barbara brings to this book a perspective that is both compassionate and empowering. Dr. Barbara's approach to health is holistic, grounded in the belief that true wellness encompasses not just the physical body but the mind and spirit as well. Her method, refined over years of working with patients and natural remedies, encourages us to look beyond isolated symptoms and instead seek balance and harmony within. Dr. Barbara doesn't simply prescribe remedies; she invites us to understand our bodies on a deeper level, to see each ache or imbalance as a message from within.

In her practice, Dr. Barbara has found that castor oil aligns beautifully with her philosophy. It's a remedy that doesn't force the body to comply but instead encourages it to heal from within. Each remedy in this book is a reflection of this belief—that the body has an innate ability to restore itself when given the right tools and support. Castor oil is one such tool. It penetrates deeply, gently urging tissues to repair, inflammation to subside, and toxins to release. It's a holistic healer, one that works with the body rather than against it, and Dr. Barbara's guidance throughout these pages is here to help you make the most of it.

In this approach, health is not a series of quick fixes or temporary solutions. Instead, it's a journey, one that invites you to understand your unique needs and rhythms. Dr. Barbara's hope is that you come to see castor oil as more than a remedy; it's a way to engage in mindful self-care, to pause and listen to your body's needs, and to honor the journey of wellness.

WHY CASTOR OIL FOR HEALTH AND WELLNESS?

In a world full of products promising instant results, castor oil offers something different: depth. It's a natural remedy that takes its time, working its way into tissues, supporting the body's natural functions rather than overpowering them. What makes castor oil stand out is its ability to provide both immediate relief and deeper healing. Applied topically, it penetrates the skin to soothe muscles, hydrate dry areas, and relieve inflammation. But beyond that, castor oil works at a root level. When used in a compress or as a gentle massage oil, it encourages lymphatic drainage, detoxification, and circulation—key processes that support long-term wellness.

Imagine using a castor oil pack on a sore back or inflamed joint. The warmth of the oil seeps in, relieving discomfort while also reducing inflammation. Over time, this isn't just about soothing pain; it's about supporting the body's own healing mechanisms, addressing the deeper imbalances that contribute to pain in the first place. Similarly, if you're dealing with dry or damaged skin, castor oil doesn't just sit on the surface; it sinks in, nourishing cells, promoting regeneration, and creating a lasting effect.

Each remedy in this book is crafted to highlight these qualities, showing you how to make castor oil a part of your wellness journey. You'll find that castor oil isn't simply a treatment; it's a catalyst for transformation, one that invites your body into a state of natural balance and resilience.

ROOT CAUSE VS. SYMPTOM RELIEF

One of the most powerful concepts Dr. Barbara brings to this book is the distinction between treating symptoms and addressing root causes. In modern health practices, there's often a focus on symptom relief—a quick fix to soothe the surface discomfort. But as many of us have experienced, this relief can be short-lived. By focusing only on symptoms, we sometimes overlook the underlying causes that lead to discomfort in the first place.

Castor oil, with its multifaceted properties, offers us the chance to go deeper. Imagine you're dealing with joint pain. A conventional approach might involve taking a pain reliever, a solution that masks the pain but doesn't address why it's happening. A castor oil remedy, on the other hand, goes to the root. It's applied directly to the area, working to reduce inflammation and improve circulation. The goal isn't just to numb the pain but to support the body's natural repair processes. Over time, this approach leads to relief that is both real and lasting.

This philosophy of addressing root causes is woven throughout this book. Every remedy is designed to do more than just bring temporary comfort. Whether you're dealing with digestive issues, skin conditions, or hormonal imbalances, castor oil offers a way to nurture your body at a foundational level. You're not simply applying a remedy; you're supporting your body's ability to heal, to find balance, and to restore itself from within.

HOW TO USE THIS BOOK

This book is more than a guide; it's a companion in your journey toward natural wellness. Each chapter is carefully organized to provide you with a clear, step-by-step path to using castor oil effectively. Whether you're completely new to natural remedies or have some experience, you'll find that each section is approachable and designed to build your confidence. Dr. Barbara has crafted this book to be both educational and practical, so you can learn and apply what you discover right away.

Feel free to start anywhere in the book. If you're looking for a solution to a specific issue, like dry skin or joint pain, go straight to that section. You'll find remedies broken down with clear instructions, so you know exactly what to do and how to get the best results. Each remedy includes tips and variations, allowing you to adjust the application to suit your needs. This structure is designed to make your experience easy, intuitive, and ultimately rewarding.

You might also want to spend time exploring the introductory chapters, which offer deeper insights into how castor oil works within the body. These chapters set the stage for understanding how each remedy fits into a broader approach to health. With this knowledge, you'll feel more connected to the process, more in tune with how each application supports your body.

NAVIGATING THE BOOK'S STRUCTURE

This book is structured to provide both guidance and flexibility. Each chapter opens with an overview of castor oil's benefits in that particular area, whether it's skincare, pain relief, or digestion. This introduction gives you context, helping you understand why and how castor oil is effective for each condition. From there, you'll find individual remedies, each one with detailed instructions that make it easy to follow along.

Dr. Barbara wanted this book to feel accessible and user-friendly, so you'll find helpful visuals, tips, and step-by-step guides throughout. Whether you're creating a castor oil pack or mixing a facial serum, the instructions are there to support you. This isn't just about following recipes; it's about building a practice, one that you can adjust and personalize as you go. The layout is intentionally simple, guiding you through each application with ease.

PERSONALIZING REMEDIES FOR YOUR UNIQUE NEEDS

One of the beautiful things about castor oil is its adaptability. Dr. Barbara encourages you to treat each remedy as a starting point rather than a strict formula. If you're drawn to a particular remedy but want to enhance its effect, feel free to modify it. Castor oil pairs wonderfully with other natural ingredients—essential oils, herbs, and other oils—each bringing its own unique properties. For instance, if you're looking to relieve stress, you might add a few drops of lavender or chamomile essential oil to your castor oil pack for a calming effect. Or, if you're focused on skin rejuvenation, combining castor oil with rosehip or jojoba oil can offer extra benefits.

This book includes suggestions for personalizing remedies so that you can truly make them your own. Experiment within the safe guidelines provided and find what works best for your body, your preferences, and your routine. Dr. Barbara's approach encourages this exploration, seeing each person's health journey as unique. By customizing your remedies, you're not only tailoring them to meet your needs; you're creating a practice that feels authentic, something that supports not only your physical health but your emotional and mental well-being as well.

BOOK 1
THE HEALING POWER OF CASTOR OIL

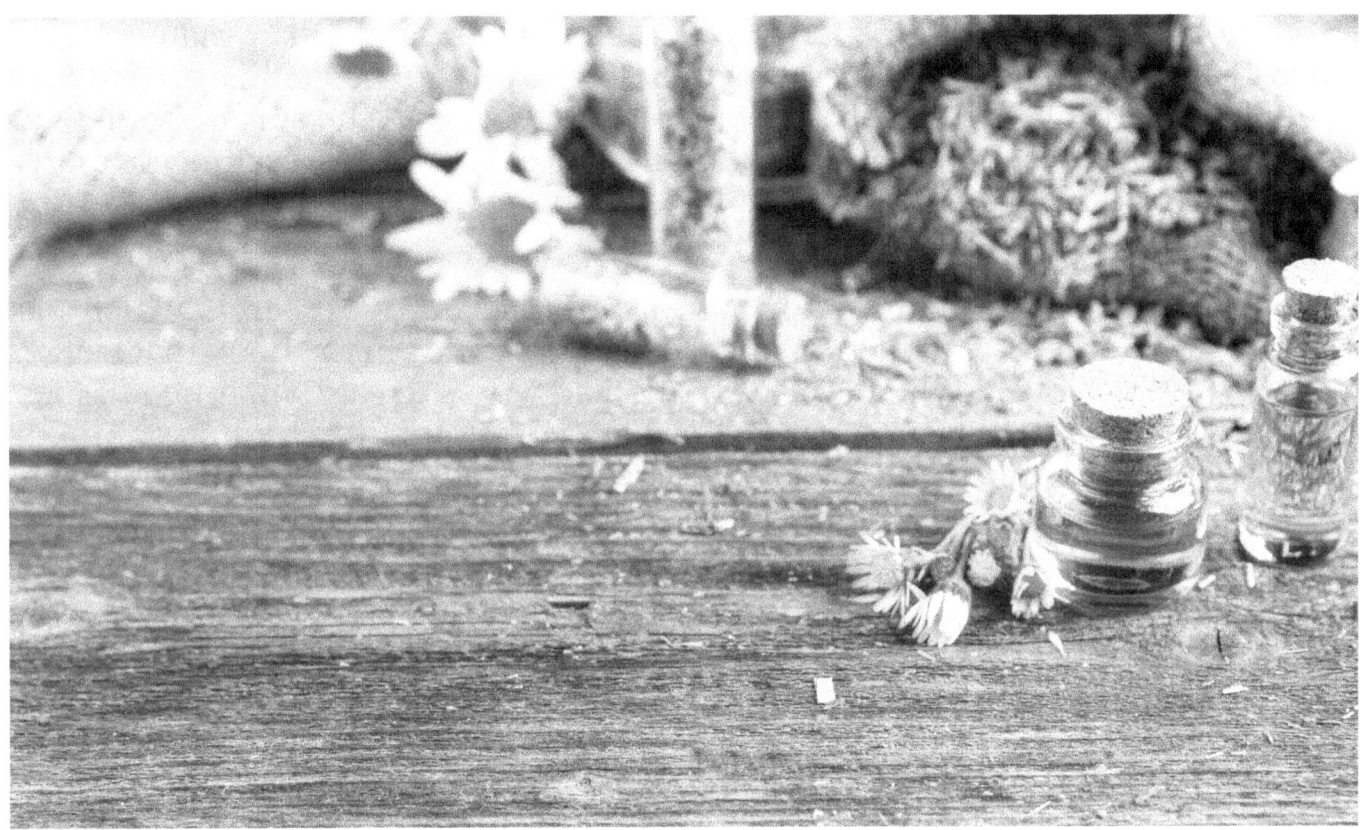

Castor oil is a unique, natural remedy that has captivated people for centuries, cherished by ancient civilizations and respected by modern practitioners alike. Its healing powers lie in its unique properties, which make it one of the most versatile oils for health and wellness. This chapter explores what makes castor oil special, highlighting the scientific and holistic qualities that set it apart. Whether applied to soothe sore muscles, nourish dry skin, or even support digestive health, castor oil works with the body to encourage natural healing from within.

UNIQUE PROPERTIES OF CASTOR OIL

Castor oil stands out among other natural oils because of its unusual composition, which gives it a wide range of healing properties. The oil is derived from the seeds of the castor plant (Ricinus communis), a resilient, hardy plant that grows in tropical regions around the world. To make castor oil, these seeds are cold-pressed to preserve the natural compounds within, creating an oil that is thick, golden, and packed with powerful nutrients.

1. High Concentration of Ricinoleic Acid

One of the key components of castor oil—and the one that accounts for many of its unique properties—is ricinoleic acid. This rare fatty acid, which makes up about 90% of castor oil, is what gives the oil its potent anti-inflammatory, antimicrobial, and analgesic (pain-relieving) effects. Ricinoleic acid is particularly adept at penetrating deep into the skin, reaching beyond the surface to deliver therapeutic benefits to muscles, joints, and tissues. This deep-reaching property makes castor oil incredibly effective for treating pain, reducing inflammation, and even fighting infections.

Ricinoleic acid's anti-inflammatory effects are backed by research, which has shown it to inhibit the production of certain compounds in the body that trigger inflammation. When applied topically, this acid works to calm inflamed tissues, which can be beneficial for everything from sore joints to irritated skin. For those suffering from chronic conditions like arthritis, castor oil offers a natural alternative to conventional pain relievers, providing relief without unwanted side effects.

2. Omega-9 Fatty Acids for Deep Moisturization

In addition to ricinoleic acid, castor oil is rich in omega-9 fatty acids, which give it its powerful moisturizing and emollient qualities. Omega-9 fatty acids, such as oleic acid, are known for their ability to nourish and soften the skin, locking in moisture and providing a protective barrier. This makes castor oil an excellent choice for people with dry or sensitive skin, as it hydrates deeply and helps to maintain the skin's natural moisture balance.

Unlike many commercial moisturizers that only coat the surface, castor oil penetrates the skin to hydrate from within. This deep moisturization is especially beneficial in dry climates, where skin can easily lose moisture. By strengthening the skin's natural barrier, castor oil helps prevent moisture loss and protects the skin from environmental stressors, such as wind and cold weather. When used regularly, castor oil promotes softer, smoother skin, reducing the appearance of fine lines and rough patches.

3. Antimicrobial and Antifungal Properties

Castor oil's antimicrobial and antifungal properties make it effective for addressing a range of skin issues, including minor infections, fungal overgrowth, and acne.

Research has shown that the ricinoleic acid in castor oil is particularly effective against common pathogens, such as Staphylococcus aureus, which is known to cause skin infections. This makes castor oil a safe, natural way to treat minor cuts, wounds, and blemishes.

For people prone to acne, castor oil offers a gentle solution that doesn't strip the skin of its natural oils. Instead, it works with the skin's own protective layer to keep bacteria at bay and prevent future breakouts. Additionally, castor oil's antifungal properties are beneficial for conditions like athlete's foot and toenail fungus, providing a natural remedy that is gentle on the skin while effectively combating infection.

4. High in Vitamin E for Skin Protection

Vitamin E is a well-known antioxidant that protects the skin from environmental damage and supports skin health. Castor oil is naturally rich in vitamin E, which helps to repair damaged skin cells, reduce signs of aging, and prevent the formation of scars. This antioxidant is especially valuable in today's world, where skin is constantly exposed to pollutants, UV rays, and other environmental stressors that can accelerate aging and lead to dull, damaged skin.

Vitamin E in castor oil acts as a shield against these factors, promoting cellular repair and encouraging the skin to retain a youthful glow. Regular application of castor oil on the skin can help reduce the appearance of scars, stretch marks, and hyperpigmentation. This makes it an ideal addition to any skincare routine, particularly for individuals looking to rejuvenate and protect their skin naturally.

5. Unique Molecular Structure for Deep Penetration

Another fascinating property of castor oil is its unique molecular structure, which allows it to penetrate deeply into the skin and underlying tissues. Unlike many other oils that remain on the skin's surface, castor oil's small molecules penetrate deeply, delivering its therapeutic compounds directly to affected areas. This deep penetration is especially beneficial for treating muscle soreness, joint pain, and inflammation at a deeper level, providing relief that is both soothing and restorative.

This quality makes castor oil a popular choice for compresses, where it can be applied with heat to enhance its penetration and effectiveness. When used in a compress, castor oil helps to increase circulation and reduce swelling, making it a go-to remedy for conditions like arthritis, muscle stiffness, and even menstrual cramps. It works with the body's natural systems, supporting detoxification by promoting lymphatic drainage and improving circulation. This not only provides relief but also enhances the body's ability to heal from within.

6. Promotes Lymphatic Drainage and Detoxification

In holistic health, castor oil is often used to support the body's detoxification processes. The oil stimulates lymphatic drainage, which is crucial for removing waste and toxins from tissues. The lymphatic system is an essential part of the immune system, and when it becomes sluggish, it can lead to a buildup of toxins, resulting in fatigue, inflammation, and other health issues. Castor oil compresses applied to areas with concentrated lymph nodes—such as the abdomen, neck, and armpits—can stimulate the flow of lymph, helping to flush out toxins and support overall wellness.

This detoxifying effect is particularly beneficial for individuals dealing with digestive issues, as castor oil helps cleanse the liver and improve digestion. Castor oil packs are commonly used in natural health practices as a gentle way to detoxify the liver, relieve constipation, and reduce bloating. By supporting the body's natural detoxification processes, castor oil offers a holistic approach to wellness that addresses root causes rather than merely alleviating symptoms.

7. A Natural Pain Reliever

For those who experience chronic pain, castor oil can be an invaluable remedy. Its anti-inflammatory and analgesic properties make it effective for reducing pain associated with a variety of conditions, including arthritis, muscle strains, and even nerve pain. The oil's ability to reach deep into the tissues makes it effective for joint and muscle pain, where it works to reduce inflammation and relax tense muscles. Many people find that regular applications of castor oil provide a natural alternative to over-the-counter pain medications.

One of the most popular ways to use castor oil for pain relief is through warm compresses or packs. By applying a warm castor oil pack to the area of pain, you can experience relief as the oil penetrates and soothes the underlying tissues. This approach is particularly helpful for those with chronic pain who want to avoid pharmaceutical interventions. With consistent use, castor oil can help manage pain naturally and improve quality of life.

8. Supports Hair and Scalp Health

In addition to its skin and health benefits, castor oil is renowned for its ability to support healthy hair and scalp. The omega-9 fatty acids and vitamin E in castor oil nourish hair follicles, strengthen hair strands, and reduce breakage, making it an excellent choice for those with brittle or thinning hair. Its antifungal properties also help keep the scalp healthy, reducing dandruff and other scalp irritations. Regular scalp massages with castor oil stimulate blood flow, which can encourage hair growth and improve the overall health of the scalp.

Castor oil's thick, viscous texture allows it to coat each strand, providing a natural protective layer that helps prevent damage from environmental factors. For those dealing with hair loss or scalp conditions, castor oil can be a valuable addition to their hair care routine, offering a natural way to nourish, strengthen, and promote growth.

EMBRACING CASTOR OIL'S UNIQUE QUALITIES

Castor oil is more than just an oil; it's a deeply nourishing, multifaceted remedy that offers a natural solution to a wide range of health and wellness needs. Each unique property of castor oil contributes to its effectiveness, making it a valuable tool in holistic health practices. From its anti-inflammatory and antibacterial qualities to its ability to hydrate, protect, and rejuvenate, castor oil has something to offer for nearly everyone.

This chapter has laid the groundwork for understanding the power of castor oil. Now, as you move into the remedies section, you'll find practical ways to apply these unique properties to improve your own health and wellness. Each remedy is designed to harness the specific qualities of castor oil, providing easy-to-follow methods that can enhance your daily routine. Whether you're looking to relieve pain, improve your skin's appearance, or support detoxification, castor oil's unique properties make it an accessible and effective choice for natural healing.

SCIENTIFIC BENEFITS OF CASTOR OIL

In recent years, castor oil has garnered considerable attention in the scientific community for its versatile therapeutic properties, many of which were already known and utilized in traditional medicine for thousands of years. Research has confirmed the healing potential of castor oil, validating its ancient use and revealing how its unique chemical composition contributes to its numerous health benefits. This section explores the scientifically-backed benefits of castor oil, shedding light on how its components work at the cellular level to alleviate inflammation, combat infection, support digestion, and even promote lymphatic drainage. From skincare to internal health, castor oil's effectiveness is well-documented, making it a natural remedy with impressive credibility.

1. Anti-Inflammatory Properties

One of the most notable scientific benefits of castor oil is its strong anti-inflammatory effect, largely due to its high concentration of ricinoleic acid. Ricinoleic acid is a rare fatty acid that comprises about 90% of castor oil, and it has been shown to inhibit the production of inflammation-causing compounds called prostaglandins. When applied topically, castor oil helps to reduce inflammation at the source, whether it's in the skin, muscles, or joints.

Studies have demonstrated that ricinoleic acid can reduce inflammation by interacting with the body's immune cells, particularly T-cells, which play a role in the inflammatory response. In individuals with arthritis or chronic joint pain, castor oil's anti-inflammatory properties make it a valuable alternative to conventional treatments. Regular application of castor oil packs or massages can help manage pain naturally, providing relief without the potential side effects of pharmaceutical drugs. For those with inflammatory skin conditions, such as eczema or psoriasis, castor oil's ability to soothe inflamed skin makes it an effective, gentle remedy.

2. Antimicrobial and Antifungal Effects

Castor oil is not only anti-inflammatory but also exhibits antimicrobial and antifungal properties, which makes it a suitable remedy for minor infections, wounds, and skin conditions. Research has shown that the ricinoleic acid in castor oil has the capacity to fight common bacterial strains such as Staphylococcus aureus and Escherichia coli, both of which are known to cause skin infections. This antimicrobial action makes castor oil an excellent choice for cleansing wounds, treating acne, and even addressing minor bacterial or fungal infections like athlete's foot.

The oil's antifungal capabilities are particularly beneficial for scalp and skin health. Castor oil's thick consistency allows it to coat affected areas, creating an environment that impedes fungal growth. This property makes it an effective remedy for fungal infections on the scalp, toenails, and other areas prone to moisture buildup. Because castor oil is gentle on the skin, it can be applied regularly to inhibit fungal overgrowth, helping to prevent and treat conditions like dandruff, ringworm, and other skin infections.

3. Skin Moisturization and Protection

Castor oil's high levels of omega-9 fatty acids make it an exceptional moisturizer. These fatty acids form a barrier on the skin, locking in moisture and preventing water loss, which is essential for maintaining healthy, hydrated skin. Scientific studies have shown that the lipids in castor oil penetrate deep into the skin, reaching layers where they can provide lasting hydration and support skin repair.

Beyond hydration, castor oil is rich in vitamin E, a powerful antioxidant known for its skin-protecting and anti-aging properties. Vitamin E helps neutralize free radicals, molecules that cause oxidative stress and contribute to skin aging. By protecting the skin from environmental damage, castor oil's antioxidants help reduce the appearance of fine lines, scars, and wrinkles, promoting a youthful, radiant complexion. For individuals with dry, sensitive, or mature skin, castor oil offers a natural alternative to commercial moisturizers, providing deep nourishment without harsh chemicals or synthetic additives.

4. Wound Healing and Scar Reduction

The use of castor oil for wound healing has been well-documented in traditional medicine, and science has provided insights into why it works so effectively. Studies suggest that castor oil promotes wound healing by enhancing cell regeneration and reducing inflammation at the site of the wound. The ricinoleic acid in castor oil not only combats infection but also aids in the repair of damaged tissue by stimulating collagen production, a key protein in the skin's structure.

When applied to wounds, castor oil helps speed up the healing process, reducing the likelihood of scar formation. For existing scars, regular application of castor oil can soften the tissue, improving its elasticity and minimizing the scar's appearance. This effect is particularly beneficial for people looking to reduce the appearance of stretch marks, surgical scars, or acne scars. Castor oil's thick, viscous nature allows it to stay on the skin longer, delivering its healing compounds directly to the affected area.

5. Digestive Health and Laxative Effect

Castor oil has long been used as a natural laxative, a benefit attributed to the presence of ricinoleic acid. When ingested in controlled amounts, castor oil stimulates the smooth muscles in the intestines, promoting bowel movements. This effect is achieved through the activation of EP3 receptors in the intestine, which increase peristalsis (the movement of the intestines), helping relieve constipation.

Although castor oil should only be used as a laxative under medical guidance due to its potency, research supports its effectiveness for treating occasional constipation. In studies comparing castor oil to other laxatives, patients who used castor oil experienced prompt relief from constipation with minimal side effects. Because it is a natural alternative, it is often preferred by those seeking non-pharmaceutical options. It's worth noting that castor oil should be used with caution and in small amounts, as larger doses can cause abdominal discomfort and cramping.

6. Enhanced Circulation and Lymphatic Drainage

Castor oil is frequently used in holistic health practices to promote circulation and lymphatic drainage. Studies have shown that castor oil packs, applied externally with heat, can improve blood flow and stimulate the lymphatic system. The lymphatic system is responsible for clearing waste and toxins from tissues, and poor lymphatic flow can contribute to swelling, fatigue, and an impaired immune response.

By supporting lymphatic drainage, castor oil helps the body's detoxification process, which can improve overall health and well-being. Research indicates that castor oil may stimulate the production of lymphocytes, immune cells that help protect the body from pathogens. Regular use of castor oil packs on areas with concentrated lymph nodes, such as the abdomen, neck, and armpits, can support a healthy immune response and reduce inflammation in the body. This practice is particularly beneficial for individuals looking to detoxify or address chronic inflammation naturally.

7. Pain Relief and Analgesic Effects

Castor oil's anti-inflammatory and analgesic properties make it effective for reducing pain and discomfort, especially for conditions like arthritis, sore muscles, and joint pain. Studies have shown that ricinoleic acid can decrease pain by modulating the release of neurotransmitters involved in pain perception. By blocking certain inflammatory compounds and stimulating local blood flow, castor oil helps to relieve pain directly at the source.

For individuals with chronic pain or inflammation, applying a warm castor oil compress can offer significant relief. Research has found that the warmth, combined with castor oil's deep-penetrating effects, enhances circulation and reduces muscle stiffness. Unlike synthetic pain relievers, castor oil provides pain relief without the risk of dependency or side effects, making it a safe, natural option for long-term use.

8. Hair Growth and Scalp Health

The scientific benefits of castor oil extend to hair and scalp health as well. Its high levels of ricinoleic acid and omega-9 fatty acids make it an effective treatment for stimulating hair growth, reducing hair loss, and maintaining a healthy scalp. Studies suggest that castor oil increases blood circulation in the scalp, which nourishes hair follicles and promotes growth. The oil's thick consistency coats each strand, protecting it from environmental damage and preventing breakage.

Castor oil's antimicrobial properties are also beneficial for individuals with dandruff or scalp infections. By reducing fungal and bacterial overgrowth, castor oil helps maintain a balanced scalp environment. Regular scalp massages with castor oil can improve overall hair health, making it thicker, shinier, and more resilient.

EMBRACING CASTOR OIL'S SCIENTIFIC BENEFITS

Castor oil's scientifically supported benefits underscore its value as a natural remedy with far-reaching applications. Its anti-inflammatory, antimicrobial, and pain-relieving properties make it an essential tool for addressing both internal and external health concerns. With its unique composition and scientifically proven effects, castor oil is not only a bridge between ancient practices and modern wellness but also a practical, powerful solution for anyone looking to embrace natural health. Whether you're using it for skin, pain relief, hair care, or digestion, castor oil offers a safe, effective, and scientifically validated approach to holistic health.

REMEDIES FOR CASTOR OIL APPLICATIONS

Each of the following remedies is crafted to make the most of castor oil's unique therapeutic properties, providing relief and nourishment for specific needs. These recipes are simple, effective, and customizable, allowing you to adapt them based on your preferences or specific requirements. Use these remedies as part of your natural wellness routine, adding the healing benefits of castor oil to your daily life.

1. Castor Oil Healing Salve

Purpose: Ideal for treating cuts, scrapes, and minor skin irritations, this salve provides soothing relief and promotes faster healing. The antimicrobial properties of castor oil help keep wounds clean, while the fatty acids aid in tissue repair.

INGREDIENTS

- 1/4 cup castor oil
- 2 tablespoons beeswax
- 1 tablespoon coconut oil
- 5 drops tea tree oil (optional, for extra antimicrobial effects)

1. Instructions
2. Melt the beeswax and coconut oil together in a double boiler over low heat.
3. Combine the castor oil with the melted ingredients and stir thoroughly.
4. Add the tea tree oil, if desired, and mix well.
5. Pour the mixture into a small, clean jar and allow it to cool and solidify.

How to Use: Apply a small amount to cuts, scrapes, or irritated areas as needed. Store in a cool, dry place for long-lasting use.

Tip: Add lavender oil for added soothing properties and a gentle aroma.

2. Ricinoleic Acid Skin Serum

Purpose: This serum deeply nourishes, reduces inflammation, and improves overall skin texture. Perfect for those with sensitive or aging skin, it harnesses the unique properties of ricinoleic acid to deliver visible results.

INGREDIENTS

- 2 tablespoons castor oil
- 1 tablespoon rosehip seed oil (for anti-aging benefits)
- 5 drops frankincense essential oil (optional, for added skin toning)

INSTRUCTIONS

1. Combine the castor oil and rosehip seed oil in a small glass bottle with a dropper.
2. Add the frankincense oil if desired, then shake well to blend.

How to Use: Apply 2-3 drops to clean skin at night, gently massaging it into the face and neck.

Tip: Adjust the ratio by adding a few drops of jojoba or argan oil if you prefer a lighter serum for daytime use.

3. Moisturizing Body Balm

Purpose: This luxurious body balm hydrates deeply and promotes skin elasticity. Ideal for dry or rough skin, it creates a protective layer that locks in moisture and keeps skin soft.

INGREDIENTS

- 1/4 cup castor oil
- 1/4 cup shea butter
- 2 tablespoons cocoa butter
- 5 drops vanilla or lavender essential oil (optional, for scent)

INSTRUCTIONS

1. Melt the shea butter and cocoa butter in a double boiler over low heat.
2. Mix in the castor oil and stir thoroughly until fully combined.
3. Add your essential oil of choice, if desired.
4. Pour into a jar and let it cool.

How to Use: Apply liberally to dry skin areas like elbows, knees, and heels, massaging in until fully absorbed.

Tip: Keep this balm in a cool, dry place. For a cooling effect, add a few drops of peppermint essential oil.

4. Scar Healing Solution

Purpose: This solution promotes skin regeneration and reduces the appearance of scars. Ricinoleic acid and additional oils work together to soften scar tissue and support healing.

INGREDIENTS

- 2 tablespoons castor oil
- 1 tablespoon jojoba oil
- 3 drops helichrysum essential oil (known for scar-reducing properties)

INSTRUCTIONS

1. Combine the castor oil, jojoba oil, and helichrysum oil in a small bottle.
2. Shake well to blend.

How to Use: Apply a few drops to the scarred area twice daily, massaging in a circular motion.

Tip: Add a few drops of vitamin E oil to boost healing and nourish the skin further.

5. Burn Relief Ointment

Purpose: This ointment soothes minor burns, reducing inflammation and promoting quick recovery.

INGREDIENTS
- 1 tablespoon castor oil
- 1 tablespoon aloe vera gel
- 2 drops lavender essential oil (optional, for additional soothing)

INSTRUCTIONS
1. Mix the castor oil and aloe vera gel in a small bowl.
2. Add lavender essential oil if desired, stirring until well blended.

How to Use: Gently apply a thin layer to the burn and allow it to absorb. Reapply as needed throughout the day.

Tip: Store in the refrigerator for a cooling sensation that soothes burns even more effectively.

6. Castor Oil Eye Serum

Purpose: This gentle serum hydrates and reduces fine lines around the delicate eye area. The fatty acids in castor oil improve skin elasticity, making it ideal for evening use.

INGREDIENTS
- 1 tablespoon castor oil
- 1 tablespoon almond oil
- 1 drop rose essential oil (optional, for added nourishment)

INSTRUCTIONS
1. Combine all ingredients in a small dropper bottle.
2. Shake to mix thoroughly.

How to Use: Apply a drop under each eye, patting gently with your fingertip. Avoid getting too close to the lash line.

Tip: Swap almond oil with jojoba oil if you have sensitive skin.

7. Lip Repair Balm

Purpose: This balm softens and heals chapped lips, providing a barrier that locks in moisture and prevents cracking.

INGREDIENTS
- 1 tablespoon castor oil
- 1 tablespoon coconut oil
- 1 teaspoon beeswax

INSTRUCTIONS
1. Melt the beeswax and coconut oil in a double boiler.
2. Mix in the castor oil and stir well.
3. Pour into a small container and allow it to cool.

How to Use: Apply to lips as often as needed, particularly in dry or cold weather.

Tip: Add a drop of peppermint essential oil for a refreshing, cooling effect.

8. Castor Oil Compress for Soreness

Purpose: A warm castor oil compress relieves muscle or joint soreness, promoting circulation and reducing inflammation.

INGREDIENTS

- 2 tablespoons castor oil
- Cotton cloth or flannel
- Heating pad or warm towel

INSTRUCTIONS

1. Warm the castor oil slightly and soak the cloth in it.
2. Place the cloth on the sore area, covering with the heating pad or warm towel.
3. Leave the compress on for 20-30 minutes.

How to Use: Use as needed after physical activity or for muscle stiffness.

Tip: Add a few drops of eucalyptus or peppermint oil for a cooling sensation and added relief.

9. Soothing Skin Balm

Purpose: This balm is ideal for irritated, red, or inflamed skin, providing relief while locking in moisture.

INGREDIENTS

- 2 tablespoons castor oil
- 1 tablespoon shea butter
- 1 teaspoon calendula oil (for additional soothing properties)

INSTRUCTIONS

1. Melt the shea butter in a double boiler.
2. Mix in the castor and calendula oils, stirring until well combined.
3. Pour into a jar and allow it to cool.

How to Use: Apply as needed to irritated or inflamed areas, gently massaging it into the skin.

Tip: For extra cooling, store in the refrigerator and use on sunburns or irritated skin.

10. Hand Hydration Cream

Purpose: This cream is designed to deeply moisturize and protect hands, especially useful for those with dry or cracked skin.

INGREDIENTS

- 2 tablespoons castor oil
- 2 tablespoons shea butter
- 1 tablespoon jojoba oil
- 3 drops lavender essential oil (optional, for added softness)

INSTRUCTIONS

1. Melt the shea butter in a double boiler.
2. Combine the castor oil and jojoba oil, stirring until fully mixed.
3. Add lavender essential oil and stir thoroughly.
4. Pour into a jar and let it cool.

How to Use: Apply a small amount to hands and massage until absorbed, especially before bed for overnight hydration.

Tip: For an intensive hand treatment, apply a thicker layer and wear cotton gloves overnight.

BOOK 2
SKIN HEALTH AND ANTI-AGING

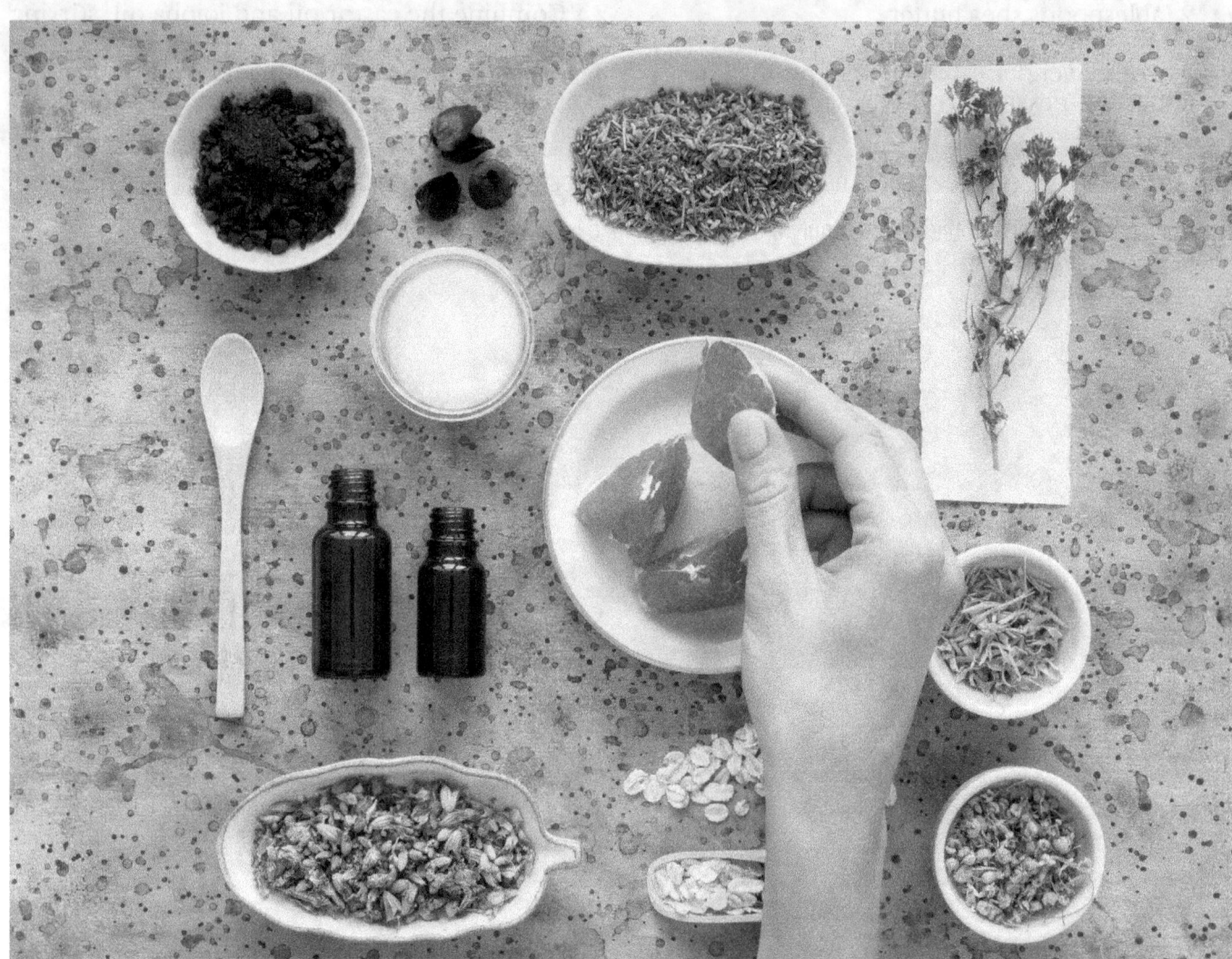

Castor oil is an extraordinary addition to any skincare routine, offering a natural way to achieve a radiant, youthful complexion while addressing common skin concerns. Rich in essential fatty acids, antioxidants, and vitamin E, castor oil provides hydration, enhances elasticity, and reduces inflammation, making it an ideal choice for anti-aging and overall skin health. In this chapter, you'll discover how to incorporate castor oil into your daily skincare routine, understand its anti-aging benefits, and explore a variety of remedies that can bring you closer to the glowing, smooth skin you desire.

DAILY SKIN CARE ROUTINE

A consistent and effective skincare routine can transform the look and feel of your skin. Castor oil's versatility makes it a fantastic base for many skincare practices, from cleansing and moisturizing to addressing specific skin issues. With the right routine, you can make the most of castor oil's natural properties, achieving healthy, balanced skin without relying on synthetic ingredients.

A solid daily routine with castor oil begins with cleansing. Castor oil's unique ability to penetrate deeply into the skin allows it to lift dirt, impurities, and excess oil, making it an excellent choice for oil cleansing. Unlike harsh cleansers that strip the skin of natural oils, castor oil respects the skin's natural barrier, leaving it soft and hydrated. To use castor oil as a cleanser, apply a small amount to dry skin, massage in circular motions, and wipe away with a warm, damp cloth.

After cleansing, toning helps to balance the skin's pH and prepare it for moisturization. While castor oil is not a toner itself, using a gentle, alcohol-free toner that complements castor oil can help tighten pores and provide additional hydration. For an added glow, consider mixing a few drops of castor oil with a toner to create a lightweight, hydrating mist.

Moisturizing is crucial for maintaining skin elasticity and hydration. Castor oil's fatty acids lock in moisture, making it an excellent standalone moisturizer or as an ingredient in creams. If you prefer a lighter feel, mix castor oil with a carrier oil like jojoba or argan oil, which will still provide deep hydration but with a less viscous texture. Massage a small amount into the skin, focusing on areas prone to dryness or wrinkles.

For nighttime, consider adding a few extra steps to your skincare regimen. Applying a castor oil-based serum with anti-aging properties before bed can work wonders while your skin undergoes its natural repair process. Regular use of castor oil in this way keeps skin smooth, supple, and radiant.

ANTI-AGING BENEFITS

Castor oil is often called a "miracle oil" in anti-aging skincare because of its ability to target multiple aging factors simultaneously. Aging skin typically loses moisture, elasticity, and firmness due to a decline in collagen and elastin production. External factors like UV rays, pollution, and free radicals further accelerate this process, leading to wrinkles, fine lines, and pigmentation. Castor oil's natural composition counters these effects, offering a holistic approach to maintaining youthful skin.

One of castor oil's most powerful anti-aging components is ricinoleic acid, which has potent anti-inflammatory properties. Inflammation is one of the underlying causes of skin aging, contributing to a breakdown in collagen and accelerating wrinkle formation. By reducing inflammation, castor oil preserves the skin's structure and helps maintain a smooth, firm appearance.

Additionally, castor oil's rich antioxidant content protects the skin from oxidative stress. Antioxidants neutralize free radicals—unstable molecules that damage skin cells and lead to visible signs of aging. Vitamin E in castor oil provides a double benefit by both protecting and repairing the skin, helping to fade dark spots and prevent new ones from forming.

The deeply hydrating nature of castor oil keeps skin plump and elastic. Hydrated skin appears more youthful and less prone to wrinkles. The oil's fatty acids penetrate deep into the skin layers, delivering hydration where it's needed most. This deep moisturizing effect not only enhances skin texture but also reduces the appearance of fine lines.

Over time, consistent application of castor oil can lead to noticeable improvements in skin tone, texture, and elasticity. Its ability to boost collagen production further supports skin firmness, making it a favorite for those looking to achieve anti-aging effects without chemicals or invasive treatments.

REMEDIES

The following remedies are designed to incorporate castor oil into your skincare routine, each tailored to address a specific skin concern. These recipes use simple, natural ingredients and are easy to prepare at home.

11. Anti-Aging Castor Oil Night Cream

Purpose: Reduces fine lines and wrinkles, deeply hydrates, and promotes skin repair overnight.

INGREDIENTS

- 2 tablespoons castor oil
- 1 tablespoon shea butter
- 5 drops rosehip seed oil
- 3 drops frankincense essential oil (optional, for anti-aging benefits)

INSTRUCTIONS

1. Melt the shea butter in a double boiler.
2. Combine with castor oil and rosehip seed oil, stirring well.
3. Add frankincense oil, pour into a small jar, and let cool.

How to Use: Apply a small amount to the face and neck before bed, massaging gently.

12. Acne Scar Healing Mask

Purpose: Reduces acne scars and promotes an even skin tone.

INGREDIENTS
- 1 tablespoon castor oil
- 1 tablespoon honey
- 1/2 teaspoon lemon juice (optional, for lightening scars)

INSTRUCTIONS
1. Mix all ingredients in a bowl.
2. Apply to the face, focusing on scarred areas.

How to Use: Leave on for 15 minutes, then rinse off. Use once a week.

13. Dark Spot Correcting Serum

Purpose: Fades dark spots and hyperpigmentation.

INGREDIENTS
- 1 tablespoon castor oil
- 1/2 tablespoon jojoba oil
- 3 drops vitamin C serum

INSTRUCTIONS
1. Combine all ingredients in a dropper bottle.
2. Shake well before each use.

How to Use: Apply a few drops to dark spots, gently massaging in.

14. Castor Oil and Turmeric Brightening Mask

Purpose: Brightens skin and evens out skin tone.

INGREDIENTS
- 1 tablespoon castor oil
- 1 teaspoon turmeric powder
- 1 tablespoon yogurt (optional, for a cooling effect)

INSTRUCTIONS
1. Mix all ingredients into a paste.
2. Apply an even layer to the face.

How to Use: Leave on for 10-15 minutes, then rinse thoroughly.

15. Fine Line Smoothing Cream

Purpose: Smooths fine lines and hydrates dry areas.

INGREDIENTS

- 1 tablespoon castor oil
- 1 tablespoon aloe vera gel
- 3 drops carrot seed oil

INSTRUCTIONS

1. Mix all ingredients in a small container.
2. Stir until smooth.

How to Use: Apply to areas with fine lines, like around the mouth and eyes.

16. Skin Firming Lotion

Purpose: Enhances skin elasticity and firmness.

INGREDIENTS

- 1/4 cup castor oil
- 1/4 cup cocoa butter
- 5 drops rosemary essential oil

INSTRUCTIONS

1. Melt cocoa butter, then mix with castor oil and rosemary oil.
2. Stir well and pour into a jar.

How to Use: Apply daily to areas needing firmness, like the neck or décolletage.

17. Castor Oil Makeup Remover

Purpose: Gently removes makeup while nourishing the skin.

INGREDIENTS

- 2 tablespoons castor oil
- 2 tablespoons olive oil

INSTRUCTIONS

1. Mix both oils in a small bottle.
2. Shake well before use.

How to Use: Apply with a cotton pad to remove makeup, then rinse.

18. Deep Pore Cleansing Oil

Purpose: Cleanses pores deeply, removing impurities and excess oils.

INGREDIENTS
- 1 tablespoon castor oil
- 1 tablespoon grapeseed oil

INSTRUCTIONS
1. Combine oils in a bottle.
2. Shake well before each use.

How to Use: Massage onto the face and rinse with warm water.

19. Wrinkle-Reducing Eye Cream

Purpose: Hydrates and reduces fine lines around the eyes.

INGREDIENTS
- 1 tablespoon castor oil
- 1 tablespoon almond oil
- 1 drop rose essential oil

INSTRUCTIONS
1. Mix oils in a dropper bottle.

How to Use: Apply a drop under each eye at night.

20. Castor Oil Face Glow Serum

Purpose: Enhances glow and rejuvenates tired skin.

INGREDIENTS
- 1 tablespoon castor oil
- 1/2 tablespoon rosehip oil

INSTRUCTIONS
1. Mix in a dropper bottle.

How to Use: Massage a few drops into clean skin.

21. Hydrating Face Mist

Purpose: Refreshes and hydrates throughout the day.

INGREDIENTS
- 1 cup rose water
- 5 drops castor oil

INSTRUCTIONS
1. Combine in a spray bottle.

How to Use: Mist face as needed.

22. Skin Detoxifying Mask

Purpose: Draws out impurities and detoxifies skin.

INGREDIENTS
- 1 tablespoon castor oil
- 1 tablespoon bentonite clay

INSTRUCTIONS
1. Mix into a paste.

How to Use: Apply for 10 minutes and rinse.

23. Under Eye Dark Circle Balm

Purpose: Reduces dark circles and hydrates the eye area.

INGREDIENTS
- 1 tablespoon castor oil
- 1/2 teaspoon vitamin E oil

INSTRUCTIONS
1. Mix oils in a small container.

How to Use: Dab lightly under eyes before bed.

24. Oil-Free Moisturizer

Purpose: Provides lightweight hydration for oily skin.

INGREDIENTS
- 1 tablespoon aloe vera gel
- 3 drops castor oil

INSTRUCTIONS
1. Mix well in a small jar.

How to Use: Apply to face as a light moisturizer.

25. Pigmentation Reduction Oil

Purpose: Fades pigmentation and evens skin tone.

INGREDIENTS
- 1 tablespoon castor oil
- 5 drops lemon essential oil (optional)

INSTRUCTIONS
1. Combine in a dropper bottle.

How to Use: Apply to pigmented areas at night.

BOOK 3
HAIR AND SCALP WELLNESS

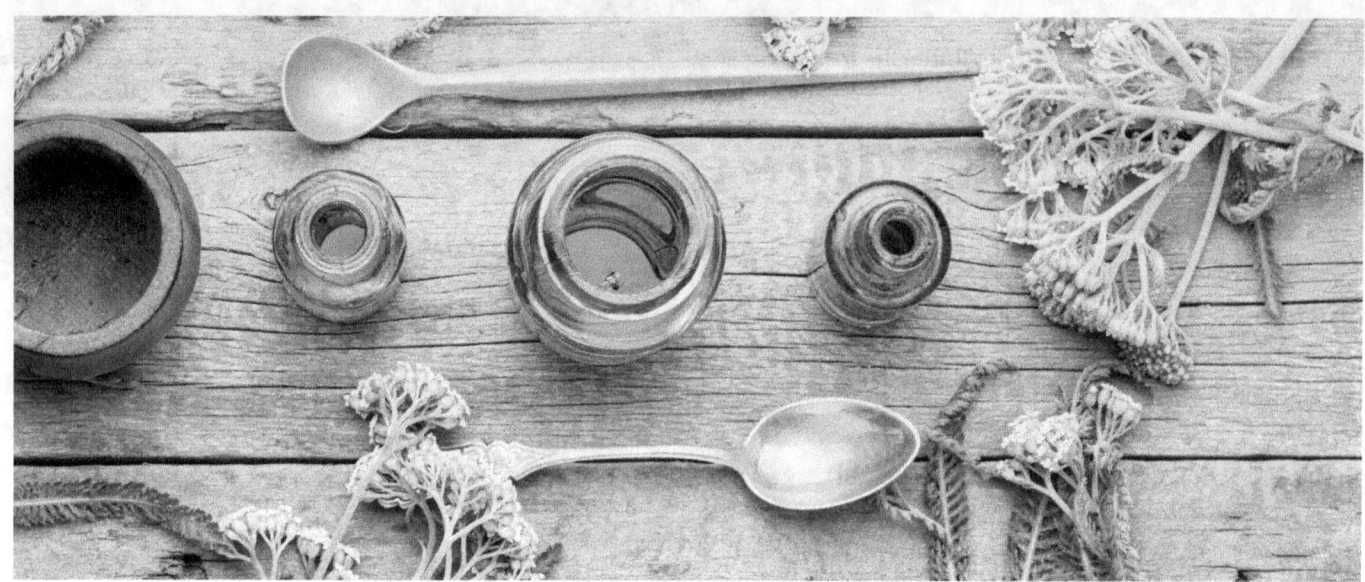

Healthy, vibrant hair and a well-nourished scalp are achievable with natural remedies, and castor oil stands out as an exceptional ingredient for promoting hair growth, enhancing hair texture, and addressing scalp concerns. Rich in ricinoleic acid, omega-9 fatty acids, and vitamin E, castor oil penetrates deeply to moisturize the scalp, repair damaged hair, and stimulate hair follicles. In this chapter, we'll explore how castor oil can support your journey to achieving stronger, healthier hair, and address common scalp issues.

HAIR GROWTH AND NOURISHMENT

Hair health is largely dependent on the health of the scalp and the strength of individual hair follicles. Factors like stress, diet, environmental pollutants, and frequent use of styling tools can damage the scalp and weaken hair. Castor oil offers a natural solution, with its high concentration of ricinoleic acid stimulating blood circulation in the scalp. Improved circulation nourishes hair follicles, allowing them to grow stronger, thicker hair.

Using castor oil consistently can result in fuller, more resilient hair. Its vitamin E content is particularly effective for hair restoration, as it aids in repairing damaged hair cells and sealing in moisture. By forming a protective layer around each strand, castor oil also reduces breakage and helps hair retain elasticity, giving it a natural, healthy shine.

Hair masks, oil treatments, and leave-in conditioners made with castor oil can add moisture and strength, addressing common issues like split ends, dullness, and hair thinning. Castor oil's emollient properties make it suitable for every hair type, from dry and curly to oily and straight. The following section provides remedies specifically crafted to promote hair growth and provide lasting nourishment.

SCALP TREATMENTS

A healthy scalp is the foundation for healthy hair. Issues like dandruff, dryness, and itching can disrupt hair growth, weaken hair, and cause discomfort. Castor oil's antifungal and antibacterial properties make it an effective treatment for scalp conditions, helping to alleviate issues caused by bacteria or fungus, such as dandruff and seborrheic dermatitis. Its thick consistency allows it to coat the scalp and lock in moisture, which is essential for a hydrated, flake-free scalp.

When applied to the scalp, castor oil not only soothes but also forms a protective layer that guards against environmental irritants and prevents moisture loss. This helps combat dryness and soothes inflammation, providing relief to those with sensitive or irritated scalps. Regular use of castor oil in scalp treatments can enhance scalp health, support hair growth, and create an ideal environment for strong, resilient hair.

Scalp massages with castor oil can be an effective routine for stimulating hair follicles and promoting circulation. Incorporating essential oils like tea tree, rosemary, or peppermint into these treatments enhances the benefits, providing additional antimicrobial or stimulating effects. Whether used as a daily serum, a weekly mask, or an overnight treatment, castor oil-based remedies offer a holistic approach to scalp care.

REMEDIES

Below are carefully crafted remedies that utilize castor oil to promote hair growth, treat scalp issues, and improve hair texture. These natural, DIY solutions are simple to prepare and provide effective results when used consistently.

26. Hair Growth Oil Blend

Purpose: Stimulates hair follicles and supports healthy hair growth.

INGREDIENTS

- 2 tablespoons castor oil
- 1 tablespoon coconut oil
- 5 drops rosemary essential oil (for stimulation)
- 5 drops peppermint essential oil (for circulation)

INSTRUCTIONS

1. Mix all ingredients in a small glass bottle.
2. Shake well to combine.

How to Use: Massage a few drops into the scalp and let sit for at least 30 minutes before washing out. Use 2-3 times per week for best results.

27. Deep Conditioning Castor Oil Hair Mask

Purpose: Provides deep moisture, improves texture, and restores shine.

INGREDIENTS

- 2 tablespoons castor oil
- 1 tablespoon honey (for added hydration)
- 1 egg yolk (for protein)

INSTRUCTIONS

1. Whisk the egg yolk in a bowl.
2. Add castor oil and honey, stirring until smooth.

How to Use: Apply to damp hair from roots to tips, cover with a shower cap, and leave for 30 minutes. Rinse with cool water and shampoo as usual.

28. Anti-Dandruff Scalp Treatment

Purpose: Reduces dandruff, soothes irritation, and prevents flaking.

INGREDIENTS

- 2 tablespoons castor oil
- 1 tablespoon apple cider vinegar (for balancing pH)
- 5 drops tea tree oil (antifungal)

INSTRUCTIONS

1. Mix all ingredients in a bowl.
2. Stir until well-blended.

How to Use: Massage into the scalp and leave on for 15-20 minutes before washing. Repeat weekly.

29. Dry Scalp Hydration Serum

Purpose: Hydrates the scalp, preventing itchiness and dryness.

INGREDIENTS
- 1 tablespoon castor oil
- 1 tablespoon jojoba oil (for lightweight hydration)

INSTRUCTIONS
1. Combine oils in a dropper bottle.
2. Shake to blend.

How to Use: Apply a few drops to the scalp, massaging gently. Use as needed for a hydrated, healthy scalp.

30. Castor Oil Split-End Mender

Purpose: Seals split ends and prevents further breakage.

INGREDIENTS
- 1 tablespoon castor oil
- 1 tablespoon argan oil (for nourishment)

INSTRUCTIONS
1. Mix oils in a small bowl.
2. Stir until well-blended.

How to Use: Apply to the ends of hair, focusing on split areas. Leave on for at least an hour or overnight before washing out.

31. Anti-Frizz Hair Serum

Purpose: Reduces frizz and smooths hair for a polished look.

INGREDIENTS
- 1 tablespoon castor oil
- 1 tablespoon almond oil (lightweight)

INSTRUCTIONS
1. Combine oils in a bottle.
2. Shake well.

How to Use: Apply a small amount to damp or dry hair, focusing on frizzy areas.

32. Leave-In Conditioner with Castor Oil

Purpose: Moisturizes hair and keeps it soft and manageable.

INGREDIENTS
- 2 tablespoons castor oil
- 1 tablespoon aloe vera gel

INSTRUCTIONS
1. Mix ingredients in a spray bottle.
2. Shake to blend thoroughly.

How to Use: Spritz onto damp hair, combing through for even distribution. No need to rinse out.

33. Scalp Exfoliating Treatment

Purpose: Removes dead skin cells and promotes scalp health.

INGREDIENTS
- 1 tablespoon castor oil
- 1 tablespoon sea salt (for exfoliation)

INSTRUCTIONS
1. Mix castor oil with sea salt in a bowl.
2. Stir until a paste forms.

How to Use: Apply to the scalp, massaging gently in circular motions. Rinse thoroughly and shampoo.

34. Color Protection Hair Serum

Purpose: Protects color-treated hair from fading and adds shine.

INGREDIENTS
- 1 tablespoon castor oil
- 1 tablespoon grapeseed oil (for UV protection)

INSTRUCTIONS
1. Combine oils in a bottle.
2. Shake to mix.

How to Use: Apply sparingly to damp hair, focusing on mid-lengths and ends.

35. Castor Oil Overnight Hair Treatment

Purpose: Repairs damaged hair and deeply conditions overnight.

INGREDIENTS
- 2 tablespoons castor oil

INSTRUCTIONS
1. Warm the castor oil slightly.
2. Apply to hair, focusing on dry or damaged areas.

How to Use: Leave on overnight and wash out in the morning.

36. Scalp Soothing Spray

Purpose: Provides relief to irritated or itchy scalp.

INGREDIENTS
- 1 cup rose water
- 5 drops castor oil

INSTRUCTIONS
1. Mix rose water and castor oil in a spray bottle.
2. Shake well.

How to Use: Spray onto the scalp as needed for soothing relief.

37. Hair Strengthening Serum

Purpose: Strengthens hair strands, reducing breakage.

INGREDIENTS
- 1 tablespoon castor oil
- 1 tablespoon olive oil

INSTRUCTIONS
1. Combine oils in a small bottle.
2. Shake to mix.

How to Use: Massage a few drops into the scalp and hair. Leave on for at least 20 minutes before washing.

38. Thinning Hair Support Oil

Purpose: Supports hair thickness and reduces hair loss.

INGREDIENTS

- 2 tablespoons castor oil
- 1 tablespoon black seed oil

INSTRUCTIONS

1. Mix oils in a bowl.
2. Stir well.

How to Use: Apply to the scalp and massage thoroughly. Leave on for 30 minutes before rinsing.

39. Castor Oil Hair Sealant

Purpose: Locks in moisture, giving hair a glossy finish.

INGREDIENTS

- 1 tablespoon castor oil
- 1 tablespoon argan oil

INSTRUCTIONS

1. Mix oils in a bowl.
2. Blend well.

How to Use: Apply a small amount to damp hair ends for a sleek look.

40. Hot Oil Treatment for Scalp

Purpose: Deeply conditions the scalp and promotes hair growth.

INGREDIENTS

- 2 tablespoons castor oil
- 1 tablespoon coconut oil

INSTRUCTIONS

1. Heat oils gently in a double boiler.
2. Apply to the scalp and hair, massaging well.

How to Use: Wrap hair in a warm towel and leave on for 30 minutes before washing.

BOOK 4

PAIN RELIEF AND INFLAMMATION MANAGEMENT

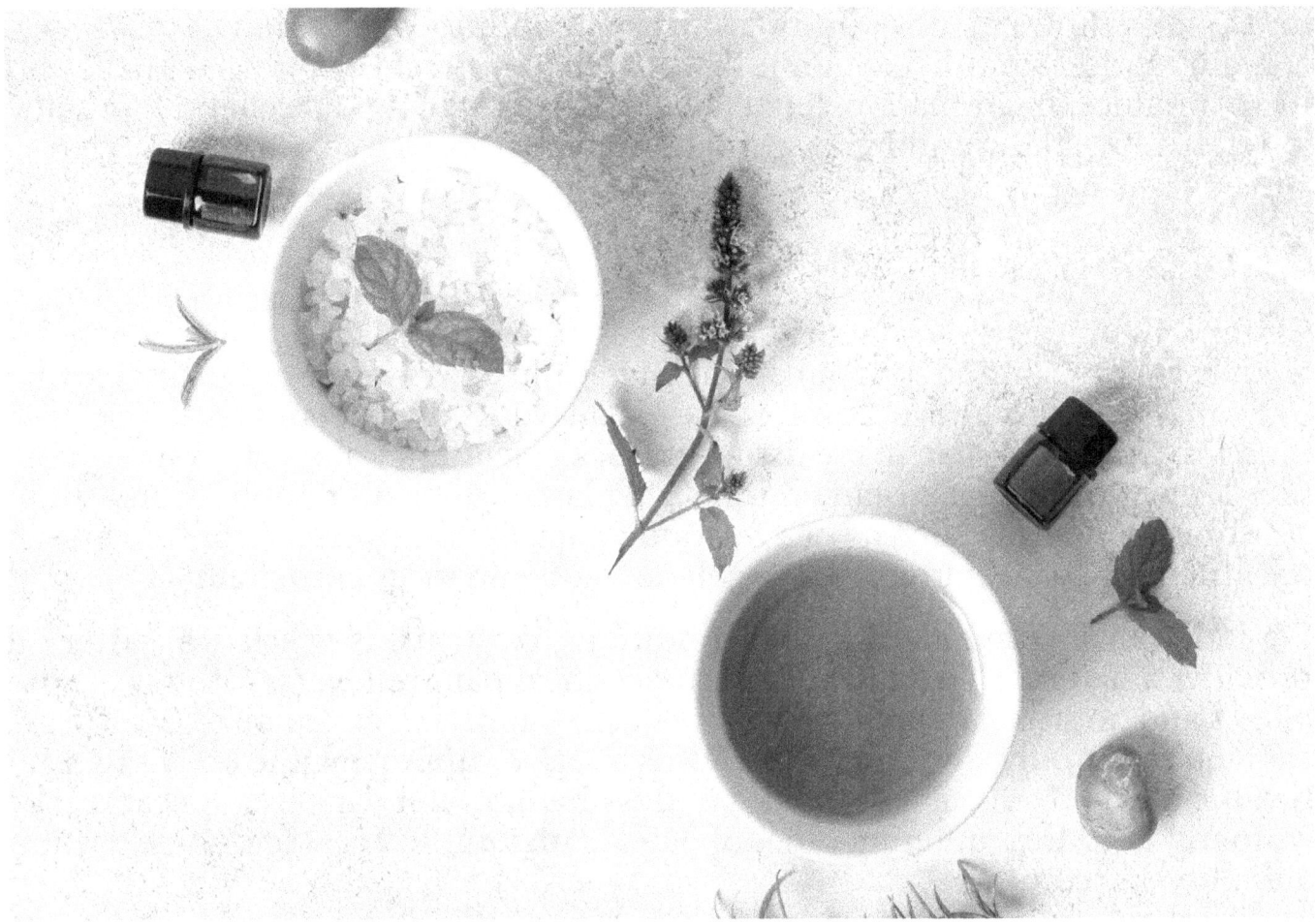

Castor oil is celebrated for its powerful anti-inflammatory properties, making it a natural choice for those seeking relief from pain and inflammation. Rich in ricinoleic acid, castor oil works on multiple levels to alleviate discomfort by penetrating deeply into tissues, improving circulation, and reducing inflammation. In this chapter, we'll delve into the benefits of castor oil for managing pain and inflammation, covering the science behind its effectiveness, and providing practical ways to use castor oil for relief. Whether you're dealing with joint pain, muscle soreness, or chronic inflammation, these remedies offer safe, natural solutions to support your body's healing process.

ANTI-INFLAMMATORY BENEFITS

Inflammation is a natural response by the body to injury or infection, but chronic inflammation can lead to pain, discomfort, and long-term health issues. Castor oil's primary component, ricinoleic acid, has been shown to have significant anti-inflammatory effects, targeting the very processes that cause pain and swelling. By modulating the body's inflammatory response, ricinoleic acid can provide relief from conditions like arthritis, tendonitis, and muscle soreness.

Studies have shown that ricinoleic acid inhibits certain inflammatory pathways, reducing the production of cytokines and prostaglandins—chemicals in the body that contribute to inflammation and pain. This makes castor oil especially effective for those dealing with chronic inflammatory conditions. Additionally, castor oil contains antioxidants like vitamin E, which help protect cells from damage and further reduce inflammation. Regular use of castor oil for pain relief can provide long-term benefits by addressing inflammation at its source.

CASTOR OIL FOR INFLAMMATION RELIEF

Castor oil's unique ability to penetrate deep into tissues is a key factor in its effectiveness for pain and inflammation relief. Unlike many topical treatments that only provide surface-level comfort, castor oil works on a deeper level, reaching muscles, joints, and even nerve tissue. Its thick consistency allows it to stay on the skin longer, providing sustained relief that lasts hours after application. When combined with heat, such as in a castor oil pack or compress, castor oil's effects are amplified, as heat improves circulation and enhances absorption.

For individuals with inflammatory conditions like arthritis or sciatica, castor oil provides a natural alternative to pharmaceutical pain relievers, with fewer side effects and no risk of dependency. By regularly applying castor oil to painful areas, you're not only alleviating symptoms but also supporting the body's natural healing mechanisms. The remedies in this chapter offer various applications of castor oil to address different types of pain, from joint stiffness to muscle tension and nerve discomfort.

PAIN RELIEF APPLICATIONS

Using castor oil for pain relief involves both direct topical application and specialized techniques like compresses and packs. Massaging castor oil into sore muscles or stiff joints can relieve tension and improve blood flow to the affected area, accelerating healing and reducing pain. Compresses and packs, which involve applying castor oil with heat, are particularly effective for chronic pain and deep-seated inflammation, as the warmth helps to soothe and relax the muscles.

The following remedies combine castor oil with other natural ingredients, such as essential oils known for their anti-inflammatory properties, to create a powerful toolkit for managing pain and inflammation. These applications are gentle enough for daily use but potent enough to provide noticeable relief, allowing you to incorporate castor oil into your pain management routine with ease.

REMEDIES

Here are some targeted castor oil remedies for pain relief and inflammation management. Each remedy is crafted to provide effective relief from various types of pain and discomfort.

41. Castor Oil Pain Relief Pack

Purpose: Alleviates pain in sore muscles and joints by reducing inflammation and improving circulation.

INGREDIENTS

- 2 tablespoons castor oil
- Cotton cloth or flannel
- Heating pad or hot water bottle

INSTRUCTIONS

1. Soak the cloth in castor oil and wring out any excess.
2. Place the cloth over the painful area and cover with a heating pad or hot water bottle.
3. Leave on for 30-45 minutes, then remove.

How to Use: Use as needed for relief from joint or muscle pain.

42. Inflammation-Reducing Massage Oil

Purpose: Reduces inflammation and pain in muscles and joints through massage, improving blood flow and relieving tension.

INGREDIENTS

- 2 tablespoons castor oil
- 1 tablespoon olive oil
- 5 drops lavender essential oil (optional, for calming)

INSTRUCTIONS

1. Combine all ingredients in a small bottle.
2. Shake well to mix.

How to Use: Massage gently into the affected area, focusing on inflamed or sore spots.

43. Joint and Muscle Pain Salve

Purpose: Provides targeted relief for joint and muscle pain, reducing stiffness and enhancing mobility.

INGREDIENTS

- 1/4 cup castor oil
- 2 tablespoons beeswax
- 5 drops eucalyptus essential oil

INSTRUCTIONS

1. Melt the beeswax in a double boiler.
2. Add castor oil and stir until combined.
3. Add eucalyptus oil, pour into a container, and let cool.

How to Use: Apply a small amount to sore joints or muscles as needed.

44. Arthritis Relief Rub

Purpose: Eases arthritis pain by reducing inflammation and soothing joints.

INGREDIENTS

- 2 tablespoons castor oil
- 1 tablespoon ginger oil (anti-inflammatory)
- 5 drops turmeric essential oil (for pain relief)

INSTRUCTIONS

1. Combine all ingredients in a small jar.
2. Stir until well-blended.

How to Use: Massage into affected joints, particularly in the morning and evening.

45. Castor Oil Pack for Sore Muscles

Purpose: Provides relief to sore, overworked muscles through a warming castor oil pack.

INGREDIENTS

- 2 tablespoons castor oil
- Cotton cloth or towel
- Heating pad

INSTRUCTIONS

1. Soak the cloth in castor oil and place over the sore muscle.
2. Cover with a heating pad and leave on for 20-30 minutes.

How to Use: Use after workouts or physically demanding activities.

46. Tendonitis Support Balm

Purpose: Reduces inflammation and pain associated with tendonitis.

INGREDIENTS
- 1 tablespoon castor oil
- 1 tablespoon arnica oil (for anti-inflammatory support)
- 1 teaspoon beeswax

INSTRUCTIONS
1. Melt beeswax, then add castor and arnica oils.
2. Stir well and pour into a small jar to cool.

How to Use: Apply to the affected tendon 1-2 times daily.

47. Nerve Pain Relief Oil

Purpose: Helps soothe nerve pain and reduce inflammation in the affected area.

INGREDIENTS
- 2 tablespoons castor oil
- 1 tablespoon St. John's Wort oil (known for nerve pain relief)

INSTRUCTIONS
1. Mix the oils in a small jar.
2. Shake well to blend.

How to Use: Massage into areas with nerve pain, such as sciatica, once daily.

48. Castor Oil Heat Pack for Back Pain

Purpose: Relieves back pain by reducing inflammation and promoting blood flow.

INGREDIENTS
- 2 tablespoons castor oil
- Warm towel or heating pad

INSTRUCTIONS
1. Rub castor oil onto the lower back.
2. Cover with a warm towel or heating pad for 30 minutes.

How to Use: Use daily until pain subsides.

49. Migraine Relief Castor Compress

Purpose: Reduces headache and migraine pain through relaxation and circulation improvement.

INGREDIENTS

- 1 tablespoon castor oil
- 1 drop peppermint oil (for cooling effect)

INSTRUCTIONS

1. Combine oils in a small bowl.
2. Apply to temples, neck, and shoulders with gentle massage.

How to Use: Use at the onset of a migraine for relief.

50. Foot Pain Relief Balm

Purpose: Soothes sore feet and reduces inflammation from conditions like plantar fasciitis.

INGREDIENTS

- 2 tablespoons castor oil
- 1 tablespoon shea butter
- 5 drops lavender essential oil

INSTRUCTIONS

1. Melt shea butter and combine with castor oil.
2. Add lavender oil, stir, and pour into a jar.

How to Use: Massage into feet, focusing on sore areas.

51. Sciatica Pain Relief Pack

Purpose: Alleviates sciatic nerve pain by reducing inflammation along the nerve pathway.

INGREDIENTS

- 2 tablespoons castor oil
- Cloth or flannel
- Heating pad

INSTRUCTIONS

1. Soak cloth in castor oil, apply to the lower back, and cover with heating pad.

How to Use: Use for 30 minutes daily as needed.

52. Castor Oil Knee Wrap

Purpose: Reduces knee pain and inflammation, especially helpful for arthritis.

INGREDIENTS
- 2 tablespoons castor oil
- Warm cloth

INSTRUCTIONS
1. Apply castor oil to the knee and cover with a warm cloth.

How to Use: Leave on for 20-30 minutes.

53. Elbow and Wrist Relief Balm

Purpose: Eases inflammation and pain in the elbows and wrists.

INGREDIENTS
- 1 tablespoon castor oil
- 1 tablespoon coconut oil

INSTRUCTIONS
1. Combine oils in a bowl.
2. Apply to elbows and wrists.

54. Tension Headache Balm

Purpose: Relieves tension headaches through targeted application on temples.

INGREDIENTS
- 1 tablespoon castor oil
- 2 drops peppermint essential oil

INSTRUCTIONS
1. Mix oils and apply to temples.

55. Sore Neck Relief Oil

Purpose: Reduces neck pain through massage and heat.

INGREDIENTS
- 2 tablespoons castor oil

INSTRUCTIONS
1. Warm oil and massage into neck, focusing on sore areas.

BOOK 5
DETOX AND DIGESTIVE HEALTH

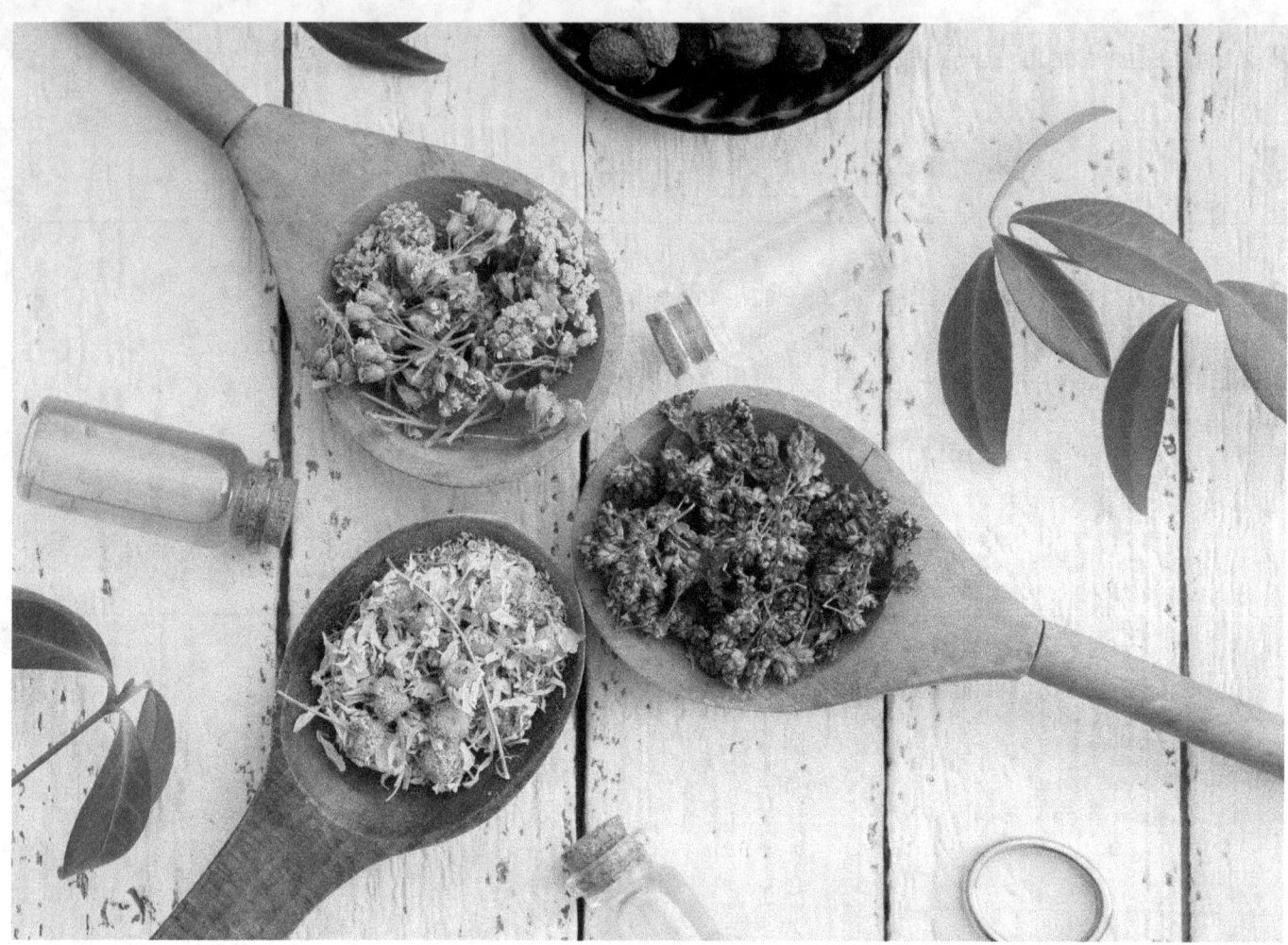

Castor oil is widely recognized for its gentle yet effective impact on digestive health and detoxification. Traditionally, castor oil has been used to support gut health, ease constipation, and promote liver function, helping to detoxify the body and improve digestion naturally. Its high ricinoleic acid content stimulates the smooth muscle lining in the intestines, supporting bowel movements and providing relief from common digestive issues. This chapter explores how castor oil can be integrated into your wellness routine to promote healthy digestion, detoxify the body, and support overall gut health.

DIGESTIVE SUPPORT

A healthy digestive system is essential for overall wellness, affecting everything from immune function to mental clarity and energy levels. Many factors, such as diet, stress, and environmental toxins, can disrupt digestive health, leading to symptoms like bloating, constipation, gas, and sluggishness. Castor oil works as a gentle aid in digestive support by stimulating bowel movements, reducing inflammation, and enhancing the body's natural detoxification processes.

When consumed in small, controlled amounts or applied externally, castor oil aids in digestive flow, relieving constipation and soothing irritated gut tissues. Its anti-inflammatory and antimicrobial properties help restore balance to the gut, improving nutrient absorption and supporting regular bowel movements. Castor oil also stimulates bile production, which is crucial for fat digestion and toxin removal, making it particularly useful for those with sluggish digestion or gallbladder issues.

BENEFITS OF CASTOR OIL FOR GUT HEALTH

Castor oil's unique properties make it an ideal natural remedy for maintaining gut health. Unlike harsh laxatives that can cause cramping and discomfort, castor oil works gently, providing a softer, gradual impact on the digestive tract. The ricinoleic acid in castor oil stimulates the gut's smooth muscle activity, encouraging movement and helping to clear out waste. This not only provides relief from constipation but also helps prevent toxin buildup, promoting a cleaner, more balanced digestive system.

Castor oil's anti-inflammatory effects can reduce irritation in the gut lining, which is beneficial for people with digestive disorders like irritable bowel syndrome (IBS) or inflammatory bowel disease (IBD). By easing inflammation, castor oil creates a more hospitable environment in the gut, allowing for improved digestion, absorption of nutrients, and reduced bloating. Regular use of castor oil for digestive health can lead to a more balanced microbiome, fostering the growth of beneficial gut bacteria and reducing the presence of harmful bacteria.

Additionally, castor oil supports liver function, which is central to detoxification and digestive health. The liver filters toxins from the blood, produces bile for digestion, and metabolizes nutrients. Castor oil packs, placed over the liver, are a popular natural therapy to stimulate liver function, improve circulation, and encourage the elimination of toxins. These packs can also relieve bloating and reduce inflammation in the abdominal area, making them a valuable tool for anyone focused on gut health and detoxification.

DR. BARBARA'S DETOX PROTOCOL

Dr. Barbara has developed a holistic detox protocol incorporating castor oil to cleanse the body naturally, promoting balanced digestion and overall wellness. Her approach emphasizes gentle methods that respect the body's rhythms and focus on restoring digestive function rather than forcing rapid elimination. Castor oil, known for its mild laxative properties, plays a key role in this protocol by helping the body remove waste without causing distress.

Dr. Barbara's detox protocol combines castor oil packs, light oral doses of castor oil, and specific dietary recommendations to encourage toxin release from the liver and colon. The protocol begins with a simple castor oil drink or smoothie taken in the morning, followed by castor oil packs applied to the liver and abdomen in the evening. During this period, Dr. Barbara encourages a diet rich in fiber, leafy greens, and hydrating foods to support the body's natural detox pathways.

By following this protocol, individuals can experience reduced bloating, increased energy, and improved mental clarity. Dr. Barbara advises doing this detox once every season, allowing the body to reset and rejuvenate naturally without harsh or invasive procedures. This gentle yet effective detox approach highlights castor oil's versatility and capacity to support long-term health and wellness.

USING CASTOR OIL FOR SAFE DETOX

Using castor oil for detox is safe when done in moderation and with an understanding of how it impacts the body. When taken internally, castor oil works as a mild laxative, stimulating bowel movements and helping to cleanse the digestive tract. Because castor oil is potent, only small amounts are recommended, and it should not be used as a daily supplement. Taking a spoonful of castor oil with warm water or herbal tea can stimulate the colon gently, making it useful for occasional constipation relief.

Castor oil packs are another effective way to support detoxification without ingestion. By applying warm castor oil to the abdomen and covering it with a heating pad, you can stimulate circulation, lymphatic drainage, and liver function. This external application helps release toxins, improve digestion, and support hormonal balance, offering a more comprehensive detoxification approach. Castor oil packs are safe for most people and can be used several times a week to support liver health and digestion.

REMEDIES

The following remedies incorporate castor oil for detoxification and digestive health. Each remedy offers a unique way to use castor oil, providing gentle yet effective relief and promoting long-term gut wellness.

56. Castor Oil Detox Drink

Purpose: Helps cleanse the digestive system and gently promotes bowel movements.

INGREDIENTS
- 1 teaspoon castor oil
- 1 cup warm water or herbal tea
- 1 tablespoon lemon juice (optional, for added cleansing)

INSTRUCTIONS
1. Mix castor oil into warm water or herbal tea.
2. Add lemon juice if desired.

How to Use: Drink in the morning on an empty stomach, but limit to once a week.

57. Gut Health Smoothie

Purpose: Supports digestion and provides nutrients for a healthy gut.

INGREDIENTS
- 1 teaspoon castor oil
- 1 cup almond milk
- 1/2 cup spinach
- 1/4 avocado
- 1/2 banana

INSTRUCTIONS
1. Combine all ingredients in a blender and blend until smooth.

How to Use: Enjoy as a morning smoothie to promote digestive health.

58. Digestive Support Tonic

Purpose: Eases digestion and supports gut health, reducing discomfort.

INGREDIENTS

- 1 teaspoon castor oil
- 1/2 teaspoon ginger powder
- 1 cup warm water

INSTRUCTIONS

1. Mix castor oil and ginger powder into warm water.
2. Stir well before drinking.

How to Use: Drink after meals for digestive support.

59. Constipation Relief Remedy

Purpose: Provides gentle relief from constipation.

INGREDIENTS

- 1 tablespoon castor oil

INSTRUCTIONS

1. Take 1 tablespoon of castor oil with warm water.

How to Use: Use only when needed, and no more than once per week.

60. Bloating Reduction Tincture

Purpose: Reduces bloating and promotes a flat stomach.

INGREDIENTS

- 1 teaspoon castor oil
- 1/4 teaspoon fennel seeds
- 1 cup warm water

INSTRUCTIONS

1. Mix castor oil into warm water.
2. Add fennel seeds and let steep for a few minutes.

How to Use: Sip slowly for relief from bloating.

61. Liver Detox Castor Pack

Purpose: Stimulates liver function and supports detoxification.

INGREDIENTS
- 2 tablespoons castor oil
- Cotton cloth or flannel
- Heating pad

INSTRUCTIONS
1. Soak the cloth in castor oil and apply to the liver area.
2. Place a heating pad on top for 30-45 minutes.

How to Use: Use 2-3 times per week as part of a detox regimen.

62. Colon Cleanse Castor Oil Drink

Purpose: Gently cleanses the colon and promotes digestive health.

INGREDIENTS
- 1 teaspoon castor oil
- 1 cup warm herbal tea

INSTRUCTIONS
1. Mix castor oil into the herbal tea.

How to Use: Drink once every 1-2 weeks to support colon health.

63. Gentle Laxative Blend

Purpose: Acts as a mild laxative to relieve occasional constipation.

INGREDIENTS
- 1 teaspoon castor oil
- 1/2 teaspoon aloe vera juice
- 1 cup warm water

INSTRUCTIONS
1. Combine ingredients in a glass.

How to Use: Drink as needed, but no more than once per week.

64. Intestinal Healing Tea

Purpose: Soothes the digestive tract and supports gut healing.

INGREDIENTS
- 1 teaspoon castor oil
- 1 cup chamomile tea

INSTRUCTIONS
1. Mix castor oil into chamomile tea.

How to Use: Drink before bed for soothing effects on the gut.

65. Stomach Soothing Castor Oil Rub

Purpose: Alleviates stomach discomfort and eases cramps.

INGREDIENTS
- 1 tablespoon castor oil
- 2 drops peppermint essential oil

INSTRUCTIONS
1. Mix oils and massage gently over the stomach.

How to Use: Use as needed for stomach cramps or bloating.

66. Digestive Enzyme Support

Purpose: Supports enzyme activity for improved digestion.

INGREDIENTS
- 1 teaspoon castor oil

INSTRUCTIONS
1. Take with a meal to aid digestion.

How to Use: Use sparingly, only as needed.

67. Natural Laxative Capsules

Purpose: Provides a convenient way to support digestion and relieve constipation.

INGREDIENTS
- 1 teaspoon castor oil
- Empty gel capsules

INSTRUCTIONS
1. Fill capsules with castor oil.

How to Use: Take 1-2 capsules as needed for digestive support.

68. Castor Oil and Ginger Tea

Purpose: Reduces bloating and soothes the stomach.

INGREDIENTS
- 1 teaspoon castor oil
- 1 cup ginger tea

INSTRUCTIONS
1. Add castor oil to ginger tea.

How to Use: Sip slowly after a meal.

69. Stomach Gas Relief Pack

Purpose: Reduces gas and bloating naturally.

INGREDIENTS
- 2 tablespoons castor oil
- Warm cloth

INSTRUCTIONS
1. Soak cloth in castor oil and place on stomach for 20 minutes.

70. Gallbladder Support Pack

Purpose: Supports gallbladder health and bile production.

INGREDIENTS
- 2 tablespoons castor oil
- Warm towel

INSTRUCTIONS
1. Place a towel soaked in castor oil over the gallbladder area for 30 minutes.

BOOK 6
HORMONAL BALANCE AND WOMEN'S HEALTH

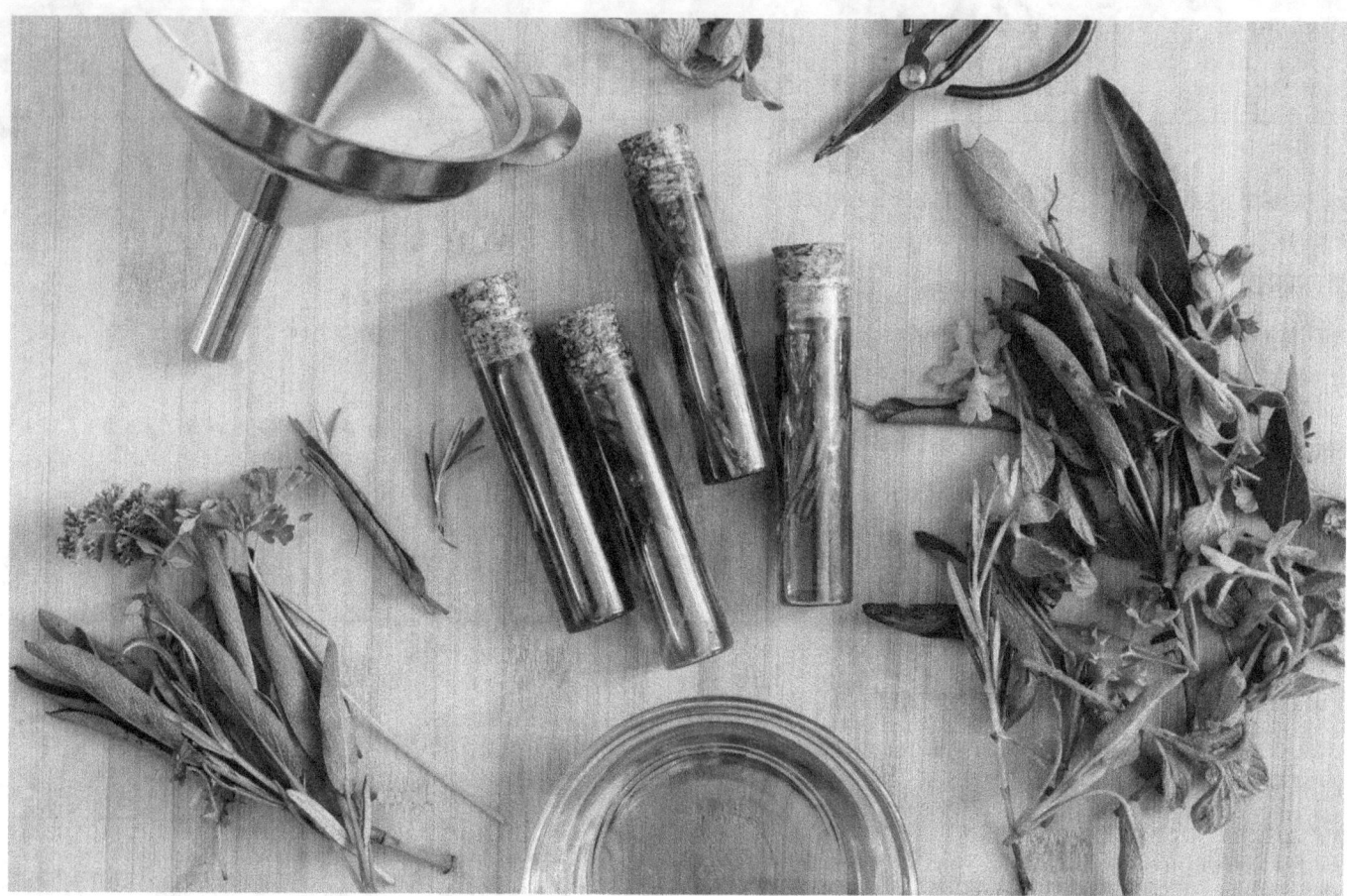

Hormonal health is crucial to women's overall well-being, affecting everything from mood and energy levels to reproductive health and skin. Hormonal imbalances can lead to a variety of symptoms, such as menstrual pain, mood swings, hot flashes, and fatigue, as well as chronic conditions like polycystic ovary syndrome (PCOS) and endometriosis. Castor oil, known for its anti-inflammatory, detoxifying, and circulation-enhancing properties, offers a natural approach to supporting hormonal balance and alleviating symptoms related to women's health. This chapter explores how castor oil can be used to manage hormonal health issues, support reproductive wellness, and provide relief from menopause, menstrual pain, and more.

HORMONE BALANCE

Hormones act as chemical messengers in the body, regulating essential functions including metabolism, mood, sleep, and reproductive health. When hormone levels fluctuate or become imbalanced, they can trigger physical and emotional symptoms that disrupt daily life. Factors such as stress, diet, lifestyle changes, and aging all impact hormonal health. Castor oil supports hormonal balance by promoting liver health, which plays a central role in hormone metabolism and detoxification. A well-functioning liver is better equipped to process excess hormones and eliminate toxins, leading to more stable hormonal levels.

The lymphatic system also plays an essential role in hormonal balance, aiding in the removal of waste and supporting immune function. Castor oil packs applied to areas with high concentrations of lymph nodes, such as the abdomen, can stimulate lymphatic drainage, reduce inflammation, and encourage the elimination of excess hormones and toxins. Regular use of castor oil packs may enhance hormonal stability by supporting liver function, detoxification, and lymphatic flow.

SUPPORTING HORMONAL HEALTH WITH CASTOR OIL

Castor oil's anti-inflammatory and circulation-boosting properties make it an excellent natural remedy for alleviating discomfort related to hormonal changes. For example, many women experience cramps, bloating, and lower abdominal pain during menstruation, which castor oil packs can help relieve by improving blood flow and reducing muscle tension. Castor oil's ability to penetrate deeply into tissues allows it to deliver benefits directly to the reproductive organs, offering relief from menstrual pain, ovarian cysts, and pelvic discomfort.

During menopause, hormonal fluctuations can lead to symptoms such as hot flashes, night sweats, mood swings, and changes in libido. Castor oil, especially when combined with essential oils like lavender or clary sage, can help ease these symptoms by reducing inflammation and promoting relaxation. Topical application of castor oil can soothe dry skin, a common menopausal symptom, and provide cooling relief for hot flashes.

For women trying to conceive, castor oil can support fertility by enhancing circulation to the reproductive organs, promoting a healthy uterine environment, and reducing inflammation in the pelvic region. While castor oil should not be used internally or during pregnancy, external applications, such as abdominal packs and massages, can create a nurturing environment for reproductive health.

WOMEN'S HEALTH APPLICATIONS

In addition to its benefits for hormonal balance, castor oil supports various aspects of women's health. Regular castor oil massages, packs, and topical treatments can be tailored to address specific issues, such as PMS symptoms, menopausal discomfort, or skin changes related to hormonal shifts. Each of the remedies in this chapter offers a targeted approach to specific women's health concerns, providing natural relief and enhancing overall well-being.

These applications incorporate essential oils and other natural ingredients that complement castor oil's benefits. Lavender, clary sage, peppermint, and frankincense essential oils, for example, are known for their calming, hormone-supporting, and anti-inflammatory effects. By combining castor oil with these essential oils, these remedies offer holistic support for a range of women's health needs, from menstrual cramps to menopausal symptoms.

MENOPAUSE AND MENSTRUAL PAIN

Menstrual pain and menopausal symptoms are two of the most common complaints in women's health. Menstrual cramps are caused by uterine contractions that help shed the uterine lining, while hormonal fluctuations during menopause can lead to hot flashes, mood swings, and other uncomfortable symptoms. Castor oil offers a natural, soothing solution for both conditions, helping to relieve pain, balance hormones, and promote relaxation.

Castor oil packs applied to the lower abdomen can reduce menstrual cramps by relaxing the muscles and improving blood flow to the reproductive organs. For menopausal symptoms, topical applications of castor oil combined with cooling essential oils can provide relief from hot flashes and night sweats. Regular use of castor oil in these ways can make a noticeable difference in managing hormonal symptoms, offering a gentle, non-invasive alternative to medication.

REMEDIES

Below are targeted remedies designed to address various aspects of hormonal balance and women's health. Each remedy incorporates castor oil for its healing properties, combined with other natural ingredients to maximize benefits.

71. Menstrual Pain Relief Castor Oil Pack

Purpose: Relieves menstrual cramps and reduces abdominal pain by improving blood flow.

INGREDIENTS

- 2 tablespoons castor oil
- Cotton cloth or flannel
- Heating pad or hot water bottle

INSTRUCTIONS

1. Soak the cloth in castor oil and wring out any excess.
2. Place the cloth over the lower abdomen and cover with a heating pad.
3. Leave on for 30-45 minutes.

How to Use: Use as needed during menstruation for cramp relief.

72. Stretch Mark Healing Oil

Purpose: Reduces the appearance of stretch marks and improves skin elasticity.

INGREDIENTS

- 1 tablespoon castor oil
- 1 tablespoon rosehip oil (for skin regeneration)
- 5 drops vitamin E oil (for healing)

INSTRUCTIONS

1. Mix all ingredients in a small bottle.
2. Shake well before each use.

How to Use: Massage into stretch marks daily.

73. Hormone-Balancing Body Lotion

Purpose: Supports hormonal balance and promotes relaxation through topical application.

INGREDIENTS

- 2 tablespoons castor oil
- 1/4 cup shea butter
- 5 drops clary sage essential oil (known for hormone balance)

INSTRUCTIONS

1. Melt shea butter in a double boiler.
2. Add castor oil and clary sage oil, stirring until well-blended.
3. Pour into a jar and let it cool.

How to Use: Apply to the body after a shower.

74. PMS Relief Massage Oil

Purpose: Eases PMS symptoms by reducing bloating and relaxing muscles.

INGREDIENTS

- 1 tablespoon castor oil
- 1 tablespoon almond oil
- 5 drops lavender essential oil

INSTRUCTIONS

1. Mix all ingredients in a small bottle.
2. Shake well before each use.

How to Use: Massage into the abdomen and lower back as needed.

75. Menopause Support Cream

Purpose: Alleviates menopausal symptoms, such as hot flashes and dry skin.

INGREDIENTS

- 2 tablespoons castor oil
- 1 tablespoon cocoa butter
- 5 drops peppermint essential oil (cooling)

INSTRUCTIONS

1. Melt cocoa butter in a double boiler.
2. Add castor oil and peppermint oil, stirring well.
3. Pour into a container and allow to cool.

How to Use: Apply to the chest and neck during hot flashes.

76. Fertility Enhancing Castor Pack

Purpose: Promotes circulation to the reproductive organs, creating a healthy environment for conception.

INGREDIENTS

- 2 tablespoons castor oil
- Cotton cloth or flannel
- Heating pad

INSTRUCTIONS

1. Soak the cloth in castor oil and place over the lower abdomen.
2. Cover with a heating pad for 30 minutes.

How to Use: Use 2-3 times a week, but avoid during menstruation.

77. Hot Flash Relief Balm

Purpose: Cools and soothes during hot flashes, providing immediate relief.

INGREDIENTS
- 1 tablespoon castor oil
- 1 tablespoon aloe vera gel
- 5 drops peppermint essential oil

INSTRUCTIONS
1. Mix all ingredients in a small jar.
2. Stir until smooth.

How to Use: Apply to the neck and wrists as needed.

78. Libido Support Massage Oil

Purpose: Enhances circulation and relaxation, supporting healthy libido.

INGREDIENTS
- 1 tablespoon castor oil
- 1 tablespoon coconut oil
- 5 drops ylang-ylang essential oil (known for its aphrodisiac properties)

INSTRUCTIONS
1. Combine oils in a bottle.
2. Shake to mix well.

How to Use: Use as a massage oil as needed.

79. Breast Health Castor Oil Pack

Purpose: Promotes lymphatic drainage and breast health.

INGREDIENTS
- 2 tablespoons castor oil
- Cotton cloth
- Heating pad

INSTRUCTIONS
1. Soak cloth in castor oil and apply to breast area.
2. Cover with a heating pad for 20 minutes.

How to Use: Use 1-2 times a week.

80. Ovarian Support Tincture

Purpose: Supports ovarian health and reduces cyst-related discomfort.

INGREDIENTS
- 1 teaspoon castor oil
- 1 cup herbal tea (like red raspberry leaf)

INSTRUCTIONS
1. Add castor oil to herbal tea.
2. Stir well.

How to Use: Drink once per week for support.

81. Perimenopause Symptom Relief Oil

Purpose: Reduces discomfort from perimenopause symptoms, including hot flashes and fatigue.

INGREDIENTS
- 1 tablespoon castor oil
- 5 drops lavender essential oil
- 3 drops geranium essential oil

INSTRUCTIONS
1. Mix all ingredients in a bottle.
2. Shake well.

How to Use: Apply to the back of the neck and shoulders.

82. Anti-Cramping Salve

Purpose: Alleviates menstrual cramps and muscle tension.

INGREDIENTS
- 2 tablespoons castor oil
- 1 tablespoon beeswax
- 5 drops marjoram essential oil (anti-spasmodic)

INSTRUCTIONS
1. Melt beeswax and combine with castor oil and marjoram oil.
2. Stir and pour into a small container.

How to Use: Apply to the abdomen during cramps.

83. PCOS Support Serum

Purpose: Supports hormonal balance and eases PCOS symptoms.

INGREDIENTS

- 1 tablespoon castor oil
- 1 tablespoon evening primrose oil

INSTRUCTIONS

1. Combine oils in a small jar.
2. Mix well.

How to Use: Massage onto the abdomen nightly.

84. Reproductive Health Tea

Purpose: Supports reproductive health and balances hormones.

INGREDIENTS

- 1 teaspoon castor oil
- 1 cup red raspberry leaf tea

INSTRUCTIONS

1. Mix castor oil into warm tea.

How to Use: Drink once a week.

85. Prenatal Skin Support Balm

Purpose: Hydrates and protects skin during pregnancy, helping to prevent stretch marks.

INGREDIENTS

- 2 tablespoons castor oil
- 2 tablespoons cocoa butter

INSTRUCTIONS

1. Melt cocoa butter and combine with castor oil.
2. Pour into a container and allow to cool.

How to Use: Apply daily to areas prone to stretching.

BOOK 7
GENTLE CARE FOR CHILDREN

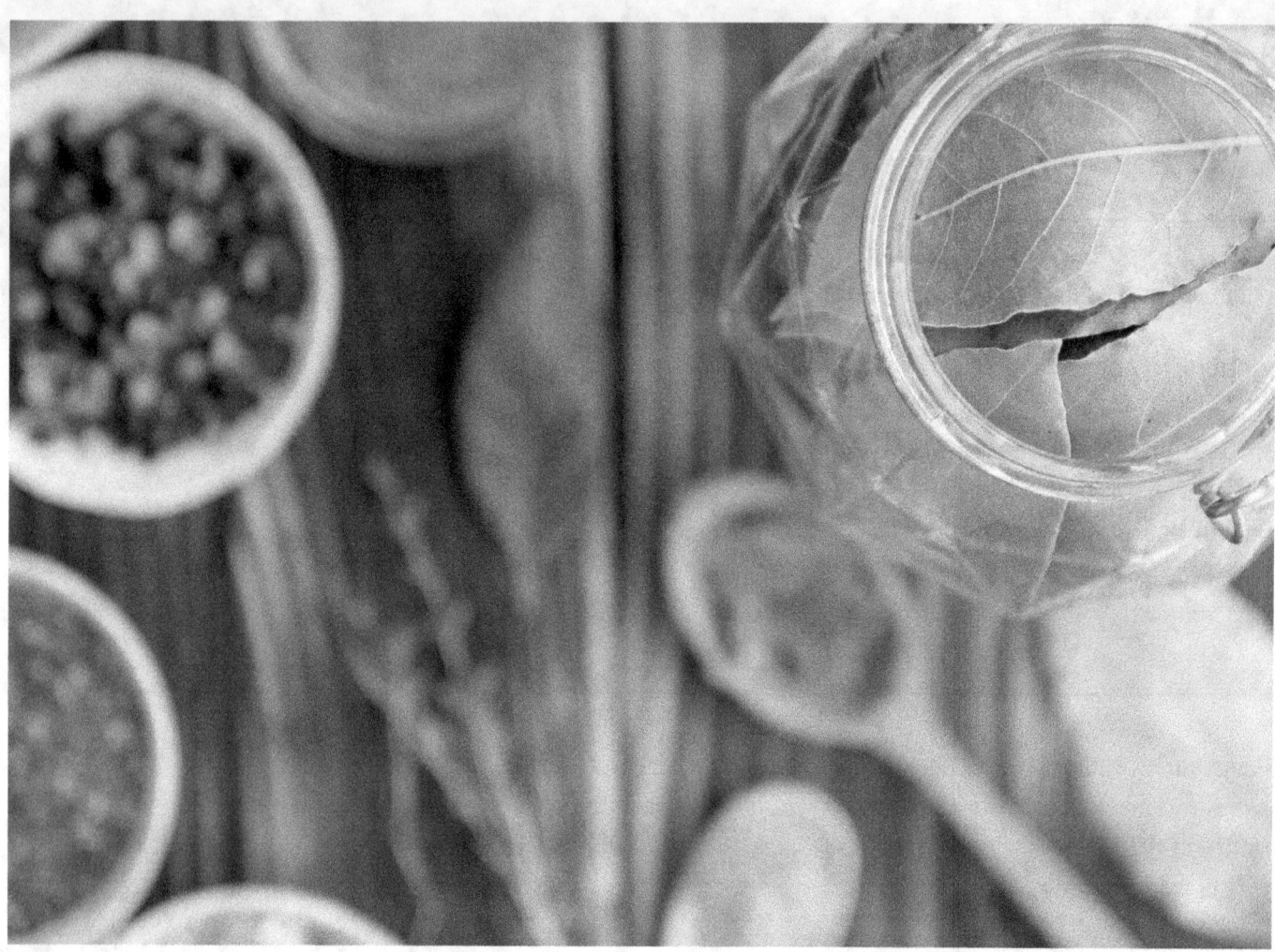

Castor oil can be a valuable addition to a child's wellness routine, offering gentle, natural remedies for common childhood ailments. Its soothing, anti-inflammatory, and antimicrobial properties make it a versatile option for skin care, immune support, and even sleep assistance. However, it's essential to use castor oil cautiously with children, ensuring that the applications are safe, mild, and suitable for their sensitive systems. In this chapter, we'll explore how castor oil can provide relief for common ailments, support immunity, and encourage restful sleep in a safe, child-friendly way.

SAFE USE FOR CHILDREN

Children's skin and bodies are more sensitive than adults', so it's essential to dilute castor oil or blend it with other gentle oils before applying. Patch testing is also advised to check for any sensitivity. For topical applications, combining castor oil with carrier oils such as coconut or almond oil reduces its thickness and makes it easier to spread on a child's skin. Castor oil should not be used internally for children, as it can be too strong for their digestive systems. Additionally, consult a healthcare provider before introducing any new remedies for children, particularly if they have specific health conditions.

For mild ailments like colds, diaper rash, and minor skin irritations, castor oil can offer gentle relief when applied externally. Using castor oil in small amounts, such as in balms or rubs, is often enough to help children feel more comfortable and supported.

CASTOR OIL FOR COMMON AILMENTS

Castor oil's soothing properties make it an effective natural remedy for common ailments in children. Its anti-inflammatory nature can calm irritated skin, while its moisturizing qualities make it ideal for diaper rash, eczema, and minor cuts. Additionally, castor oil's antibacterial properties help keep minor wounds clean, promoting faster healing. When combined with essential oils like lavender or chamomile, it provides calming effects that can be especially helpful for children dealing with colic, teething pain, or sleeplessness.

For respiratory issues, such as colds and congestion, castor oil can be used in chest rubs or compresses to open airways and ease breathing. A gentle massage with castor oil can help soothe tummy discomfort from gas or colic, while balms and lotions offer relief from rashes, bites, and other minor skin issues.

IMMUNE AND RESTFUL SLEEP SUPPORT

Building a strong immune system is essential for children, particularly during the colder months or times of stress. Castor oil can support immunity when applied topically, especially around the chest and back. Gentle immune-boosting balms, infused with essential oils like eucalyptus or tea tree (in child-safe amounts), can be applied regularly to protect and strengthen a child's natural defenses.

Castor oil can also promote restful sleep, especially when combined with calming essential oils like lavender or chamomile. A gentle foot or back massage with a sleep-support oil blend before bedtime can help soothe the child and prepare them for sleep. This ritual can become a comforting part of the bedtime routine, offering both physical relaxation and emotional reassurance.

REMEDIES

Here are castor oil remedies specifically designed for children, offering gentle relief for common issues in a safe, easy-to-use format. Each remedy uses mild, child-safe ingredients and has been crafted with sensitivity in mind.

86. Gentle Chest Rub for Colds

Purpose: Eases congestion and promotes easier breathing during colds.

INGREDIENTS
- 1 tablespoon castor oil
- 1 tablespoon coconut oil
- 1 drop eucalyptus essential oil (optional, for children over 2 years old)

INSTRUCTIONS
1. Combine all ingredients in a small container and mix well.
2. Use a small amount as a chest rub.

How to Use: Apply to the chest and back as needed to ease congestion.

87. Soothing Diaper Rash Balm

Purpose: Soothes diaper rash, calms irritation, and hydrates sensitive skin.

INGREDIENTS
- 1 tablespoon castor oil
- 1 tablespoon shea butter
- 1 tablespoon coconut oil

INSTRUCTIONS
1. Melt shea butter and coconut oil together.
2. Add castor oil and stir until well-blended.
3. Pour into a small jar and let it cool.

How to Use: Apply a thin layer to the diaper area as needed.

88. Colic Relief Massage Oil

Purpose: Reduces colic symptoms and soothes an upset tummy.

INGREDIENTS
- 1 tablespoon castor oil
- 1 tablespoon almond oil
- 1 drop chamomile essential oil (optional, for extra calming)

INSTRUCTIONS
1. Mix all ingredients in a small bottle and shake well.

How to Use: Gently massage in circular motions on the baby's tummy.

89. Mild Castor Oil Salve for Cuts

Purpose: Promotes healing of minor cuts and scrapes.

INGREDIENTS
- 1 tablespoon castor oil
- 1 teaspoon beeswax
- 1 drop tea tree essential oil (for children over 2 years)

INSTRUCTIONS
1. Melt beeswax and mix with castor oil.
2. Add tea tree oil, if desired.
3. Pour into a small jar and let cool.

How to Use: Apply a small amount to cuts and scrapes as needed.

90. Bug Bite Soother

Purpose: Reduces itching and discomfort from bug bites.

INGREDIENTS
- 1 teaspoon castor oil
- 1 teaspoon aloe vera gel

INSTRUCTIONS
1. Combine ingredients in a small jar and mix.

How to Use: Apply to bug bites as needed for itch relief.

91. Children's Tummy Relief Pack

Purpose: Eases gas, bloating, and tummy discomfort.

INGREDIENTS
- 1 teaspoon castor oil
- Warm cloth

INSTRUCTIONS
1. Rub castor oil on the child's tummy.
2. Place a warm cloth over the area for 10-15 minutes.

How to Use: Use as needed for tummy aches.

92. Sleep Support Oil Blend

Purpose: Helps children relax and sleep more easily.

INGREDIENTS

- 1 tablespoon castor oil
- 1 tablespoon almond oil
- 1 drop lavender essential oil (optional)

INSTRUCTIONS

1. Mix all ingredients in a bottle and shake well.

How to Use: Massage onto feet or back before bedtime.

93. Teething Relief Rub

Purpose: Eases gum pain during teething.

INGREDIENTS

- 1 teaspoon castor oil
- 1 drop clove essential oil (optional and very diluted)

INSTRUCTIONS

1. Mix ingredients in a small container.

How to Use: Gently massage onto gums using a clean finger. Test on a small area first.

94. Gentle Eczema Balm

Purpose: Calms irritated skin and provides moisture for eczema-prone areas.

INGREDIENTS

- 1 tablespoon castor oil
- 1 tablespoon shea butter

INSTRUCTIONS

1. Melt shea butter and add castor oil.
2. Stir and pour into a jar to set.

How to Use: Apply to affected areas 1-2 times daily.

95. Rash and Itch Relief Lotion

Purpose: Relieves rashes and itching from minor skin irritations.

INGREDIENTS
- 1 tablespoon castor oil
- 1 tablespoon aloe vera gel

INSTRUCTIONS
1. Mix ingredients in a small bottle.

How to Use: Apply to itchy or irritated areas as needed.

96. Baby Massage Oil

Purpose: Nourishes baby's skin and provides relaxation during massage.

INGREDIENTS
- 1 tablespoon castor oil
- 1 tablespoon coconut oil

INSTRUCTIONS
1. Mix oils in a bottle and shake.

How to Use: Use a small amount for a gentle, relaxing massage.

97. Children's Immune Boost Balm

Purpose: Supports immune health when applied topically.

INGREDIENTS
- 1 tablespoon castor oil
- 1 drop eucalyptus or tea tree oil (for children over 2 years)

INSTRUCTIONS
1. Mix ingredients in a small jar.

How to Use: Rub a small amount on the chest or back before bed.

98. Mild Sunburn Relief Gel

Purpose: Soothes and hydrates sunburned skin.

INGREDIENTS

- 1 tablespoon castor oil
- 1 tablespoon aloe vera gel

INSTRUCTIONS

1. Combine ingredients in a small container.

How to Use: Apply to sunburned areas for relief.

99. Earache Relief Pack

Purpose: Eases discomfort from earaches.

INGREDIENTS

- 1 teaspoon castor oil
- Warm cloth

INSTRUCTIONS

1. Rub a small amount of castor oil around the ear (not inside).
2. Place a warm cloth over the ear for comfort.

How to Use: Use as needed for earache relief.

100. Cold Relief Chest Compress

Purpose: Helps relieve congestion and ease breathing during a cold.

INGREDIENTS

- 1 tablespoon castor oil
- Warm cloth

INSTRUCTIONS

1. Rub castor oil onto the chest.
2. Place a warm cloth over the area for 10-15 minutes.

How to Use: Use as needed to relieve congestion.

BOOK 8
MEN'S HEALTH AND GROOMING

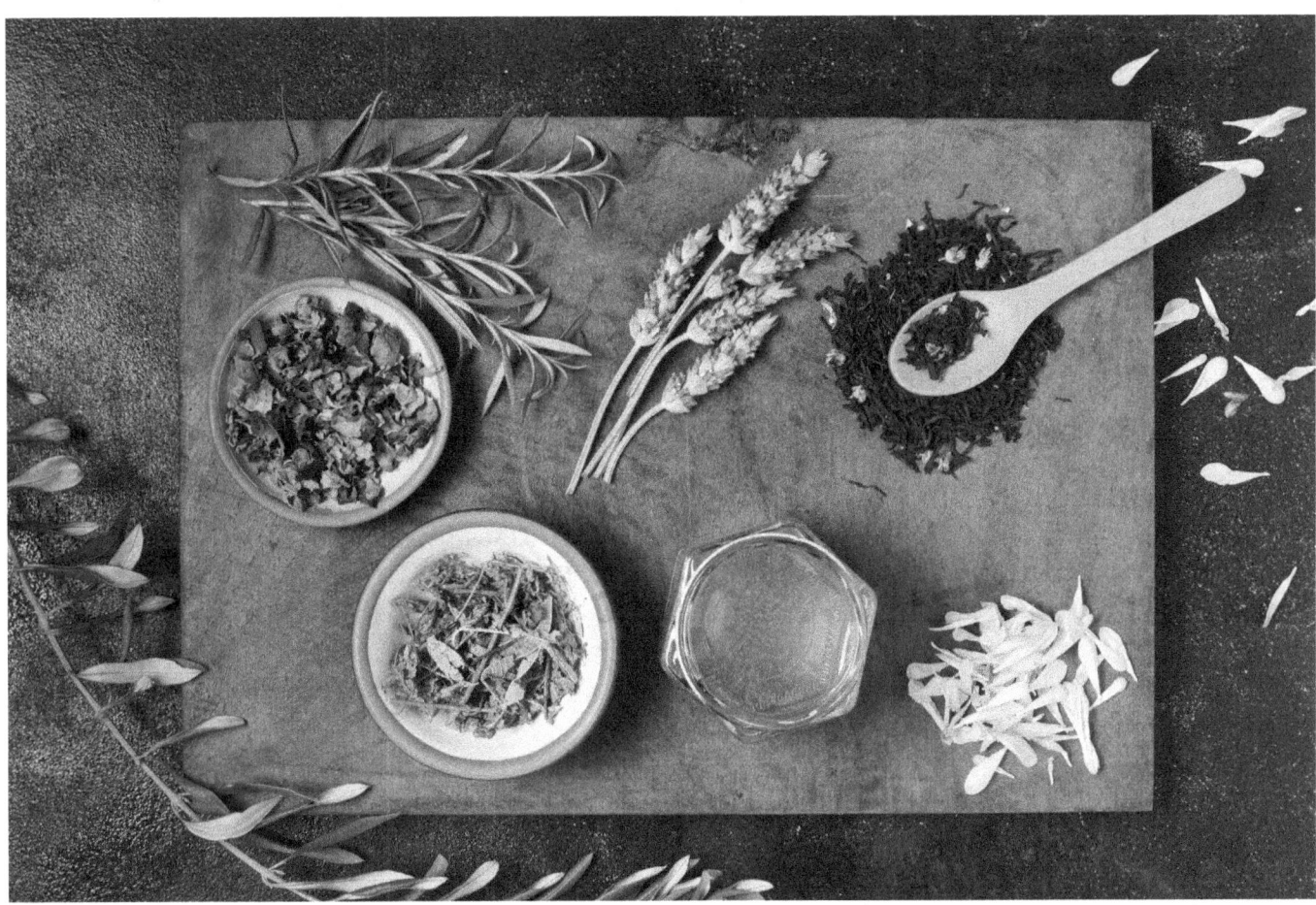

Castor oil is not just for general wellness or women's health; it has numerous applications for men's grooming, skin care, hair, and overall health. In addition to supporting skin and beard health, castor oil offers targeted benefits for muscle recovery, joint flexibility, and even prostate health. This chapter explores how men can use castor oil to enhance their grooming routines, support muscle and joint function, and maintain overall well-being. Each remedy provides a natural alternative for men seeking healthier, chemical-free solutions in their daily care.

GROOMING AND SKIN CARE

Men's grooming routines are increasingly focused on natural solutions that improve skin health and appearance without synthetic additives. Castor oil offers a simple, effective way to nourish the skin, reduce irritation from shaving, and maintain a well-groomed look. With its moisturizing and anti-inflammatory properties, castor oil is ideal for addressing issues like dryness, razor burn, and ingrown hairs.

For post-shave care, castor oil can soothe the skin, reducing redness and irritation, while also delivering moisture to prevent dryness. Its antibacterial properties help keep skin clean, especially after shaving, reducing the likelihood of breakouts and irritation. When blended with other natural oils, castor oil becomes a versatile ingredient in aftershave balms, moisturizers, and scrubs, adding a protective barrier to the skin.

CASTOR OIL FOR BEARD AND HAIR

Beard and hair care are essential components of men's grooming. Castor oil is especially beneficial for beard growth and maintenance due to its rich fatty acid content, which nourishes hair follicles, reduces breakage, and promotes healthy growth. Its thick, viscous texture makes it perfect for conditioning beards, adding shine, and taming unruly hair.

Regular application of castor oil to the beard area can also stimulate growth, making it an excellent natural remedy for men looking to achieve a fuller beard. For scalp care, castor oil provides nutrients that strengthen hair roots, reduce dandruff, and prevent thinning. Blending castor oil with essential oils like peppermint or rosemary can further enhance its effects, supporting both beard and hair health.

HEALTH SUPPORT FOR MEN

Beyond grooming, castor oil can offer support for men's health, addressing issues such as muscle soreness, joint stiffness, and prostate health. Castor oil packs, in particular, are beneficial for muscle recovery and prostate support. When applied with heat, these packs enhance circulation, reduce inflammation, and promote relaxation, which is especially useful for athletes or those experiencing muscle tension and stiffness.

Castor oil's anti-inflammatory properties make it a natural remedy for joint pain, aiding in flexibility and comfort. Applying castor oil to problem areas can provide relief from soreness after workouts, reduce stiffness, and even boost circulation, offering a holistic approach to recovery and men's health maintenance.

PROSTATE AND MUSCLE HEALTH

Prostate health is a significant concern for many men, particularly as they age. Castor oil packs applied to the lower abdomen can help improve circulation to the prostate, reduce inflammation, and promote overall wellness in the area. Regular application may help alleviate minor discomfort and maintain prostate health.

For muscle health, castor oil's ability to penetrate deeply into tissues makes it an excellent choice for muscle recovery and flexibility. When combined with essential oils such as eucalyptus or peppermint, castor oil creates a powerful muscle rub that supports faster recovery after physical activity, relaxes muscles, and aids joint flexibility. These natural solutions offer a chemical-free approach to maintaining mobility and comfort.

REMEDIES

The following remedies are tailored to address the unique grooming and health needs of men, with applications for skin, beard, muscle recovery, and overall health. Each remedy combines castor oil's beneficial properties with complementary ingredients for maximum effectiveness.

101. Beard Oil Blend

Purpose: Softens and nourishes beard hair, promoting a fuller, shinier beard.

INGREDIENTS

- 1 tablespoon castor oil
- 1 tablespoon jojoba oil
- 3 drops cedarwood essential oil (for a masculine scent)

INSTRUCTIONS

1. Combine all ingredients in a small bottle.
2. Shake well to mix.

How to Use: Apply a few drops to the beard, massaging in from root to tip.

102. Post-Shave Skin Balm

Purpose: Soothes and hydrates skin after shaving, reducing irritation.

INGREDIENTS

- 1 tablespoon castor oil
- 1 tablespoon aloe vera gel
- 2 drops lavender essential oil

INSTRUCTIONS

1. Mix all ingredients in a small container.
2. Stir until smooth.

How to Use: Apply a small amount to freshly shaved areas.

103. Hair and Scalp Strengthening Oil

Purpose: Strengthens hair follicles and reduces dandruff, promoting healthy hair growth.

INGREDIENTS

- 1 tablespoon castor oil
- 1 tablespoon olive oil
- 3 drops rosemary essential oil

INSTRUCTIONS

1. Combine oils in a small bottle and shake well.

How to Use: Massage into the scalp and leave on for 30 minutes before washing.

104. Natural Beard Softener

Purpose: Conditions and softens beard hair, reducing frizz and dryness.

INGREDIENTS

- 1 tablespoon castor oil
- 1 tablespoon coconut oil

INSTRUCTIONS

1. Melt coconut oil and mix with castor oil.
2. Pour into a small container and let it cool.

How to Use: Rub a small amount into the beard and style as usual.

105. Aftershave Moisturizing Lotion

Purpose: Hydrates and protects the skin after shaving, minimizing dryness.

INGREDIENTS
- 1 tablespoon castor oil
- 1 tablespoon shea butter

INSTRUCTIONS
1. Melt shea butter, then add castor oil.
2. Stir until well-blended.

How to Use: Apply to shaved areas for moisture and protection.

106. Muscle Recovery Rub

Purpose: Eases muscle soreness and promotes recovery after physical activity.

INGREDIENTS
- 1 tablespoon castor oil
- 1 tablespoon arnica oil (for muscle relief)
- 3 drops eucalyptus essential oil

INSTRUCTIONS
1. Combine all ingredients in a small bottle.
2. Shake well to blend.

How to Use: Massage into sore muscles after exercise.

107. Prostate Health Castor Pack

Purpose: Supports prostate health and reduces inflammation.

INGREDIENTS
- 2 tablespoons castor oil
- Cotton cloth or flannel
- Heating pad

INSTRUCTIONS
1. Soak the cloth in castor oil and place over the lower abdomen.
2. Cover with a heating pad for 30-45 minutes.

How to Use: Use 1-2 times per week for prostate support.

108. Energy Boost Massage Oil

Purpose: Enhances circulation and provides an energy boost.

INGREDIENTS

- 1 tablespoon castor oil
- 1 tablespoon almond oil
- 5 drops peppermint essential oil

INSTRUCTIONS

1. Mix all ingredients in a small bottle.

How to Use: Massage onto neck and shoulders for an energizing effect.

109. Castor Oil Rub for Joint Flexibility

Purpose: Reduces joint stiffness and supports flexibility.

INGREDIENTS

- 1 tablespoon castor oil
- 5 drops ginger essential oil (for warmth)

INSTRUCTIONS

1. Mix oils in a small container.

How to Use: Massage onto joints daily, especially before physical activity.

110. Circulation-Boosting Foot Rub

Purpose: Improves circulation and relieves tired feet.

INGREDIENTS

- 1 tablespoon castor oil
- 1 tablespoon coconut oil
- 3 drops tea tree essential oil

INSTRUCTIONS

1. Combine ingredients in a small jar.

How to Use: Massage into feet before bed.

111. Pre-Workout Warm-Up Oil

Purpose: Prepares muscles for activity and enhances flexibility.

INGREDIENTS
- 1 tablespoon castor oil
- 1 tablespoon olive oil
- 3 drops black pepper essential oil (for warming effect)

INSTRUCTIONS
1. Mix all ingredients and shake well.

How to Use: Apply to muscles and joints before exercise.

112. Beard Growth Serum

Purpose: Stimulates beard growth by nourishing hair follicles.

INGREDIENTS
- 1 tablespoon castor oil
- 1 tablespoon argan oil
- 5 drops peppermint essential oil

INSTRUCTIONS
1. Combine oils in a small bottle.

How to Use: Massage a few drops into the beard area daily.

113. Athlete's Foot Relief Balm

Purpose: Treats athlete's foot by reducing fungal infections and soothing the skin.

INGREDIENTS
- 1 tablespoon castor oil
- 1 tablespoon coconut oil
- 3 drops tea tree essential oil (antifungal)

INSTRUCTIONS
1. Mix ingredients in a small jar.

How to Use: Apply to affected areas as needed.

114. Castor Oil Face Scrub

Purpose: Exfoliates and cleanses, leaving skin smooth and refreshed.

INGREDIENTS

- 1 tablespoon castor oil
- 1 tablespoon finely ground oats (for gentle exfoliation)

INSTRUCTIONS

1. Mix ingredients into a paste.

How to Use: Gently scrub face in circular motions, then rinse.

115. Castor Oil Hair Thickening Gel

Purpose: Thickens hair and improves texture, promoting a fuller look.

INGREDIENTS

- 1 tablespoon castor oil
- 1 tablespoon aloe vera gel

INSTRUCTIONS

1. Mix castor oil with aloe vera gel in a small container.

How to Use: Apply to damp hair as a leave-in treatment.

BOOK 9
ECO-FRIENDLY HOME AND CLEANING

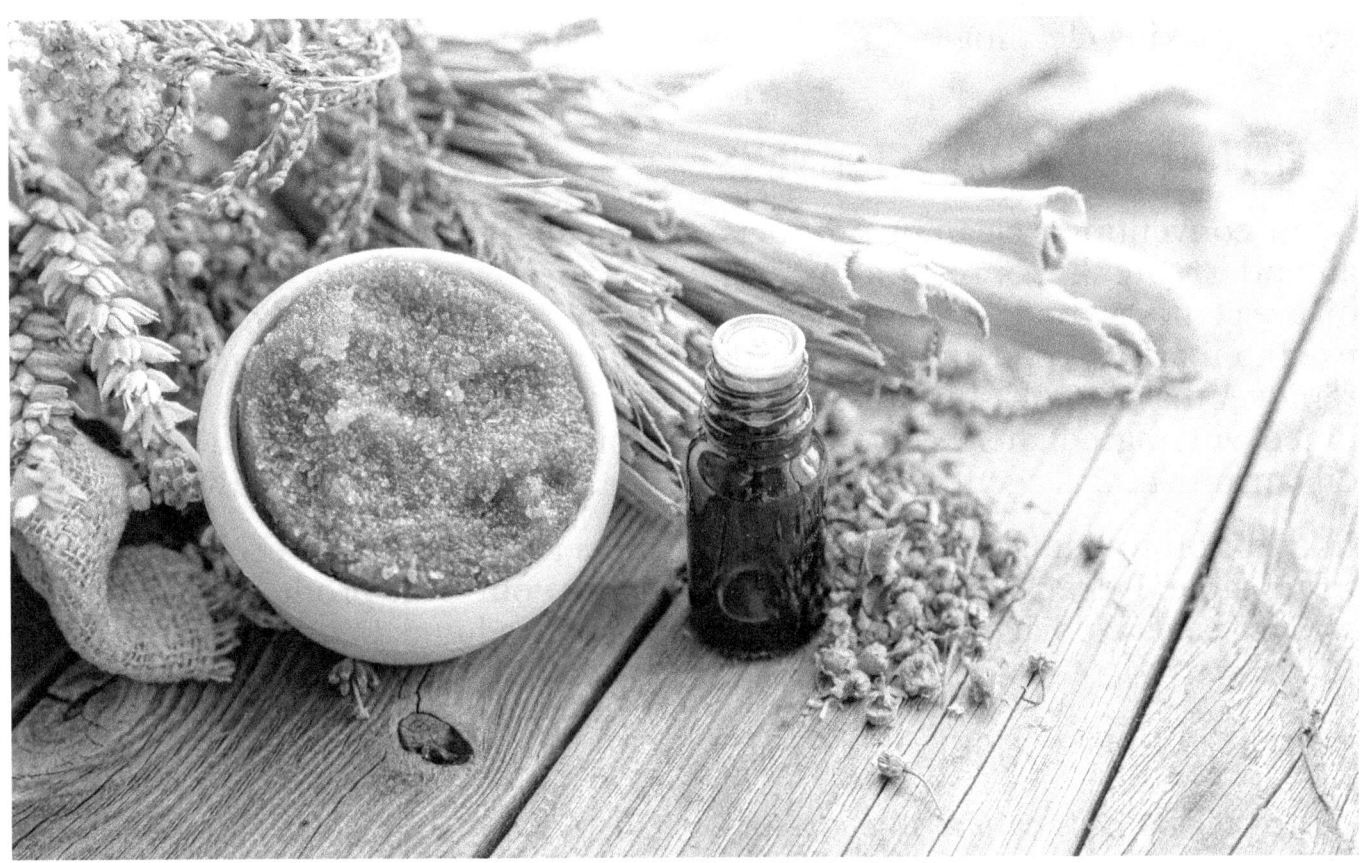

Creating a clean, healthy home environment doesn't require harsh chemicals or synthetic ingredients. Castor oil can be a valuable component in homemade, non-toxic cleaning solutions that are safe for both your family and the planet. Its antibacterial and anti-fungal properties, along with its thick consistency, make it an ideal base for a variety of household cleaners. This chapter explores how castor oil can be used to make eco-friendly cleaning products that effectively tackle dirt, grime, and bacteria without the need for harmful chemicals. From multi-purpose cleaners to specific solutions for kitchen and bathroom, these remedies can transform your home into a more sustainable, toxin-free space.

HOME CLEANING SOLUTIONS

Castor oil's natural properties make it an effective ingredient for all-purpose cleaning around the house. When blended with other natural ingredients, such as vinegar, baking soda, and essential oils, it can create powerful cleaners that are gentle on surfaces but tough on grime. Whether it's wiping down countertops, scrubbing bathroom tiles, or removing stains, castor oil-based cleaners provide a safe and effective alternative to commercial products.

Using natural cleaning solutions is especially beneficial for families with children or pets, as it reduces exposure to chemicals that can be harmful if ingested or inhaled. Castor oil's ability to blend well with essential oils also allows for pleasant scents, making cleaning feel more refreshing and less like a chore.

CREATING NON-TOXIC CLEANERS

Many conventional cleaning products contain chemicals that can pollute indoor air and irritate skin or respiratory systems. Non-toxic cleaners made with castor oil are gentle on both your home and your health. For example, castor oil can be used to make a powerful degreaser that's safe for food prep surfaces, or a mold remover that keeps bathrooms fresh and clean without harsh bleach. When combined with ingredients like lemon essential oil (a natural antibacterial) or tea tree oil (an anti-fungal agent), castor oil becomes a versatile cleaning ally.

In addition to being safer, these DIY cleaners are often more economical and sustainable. By reusing containers and mixing your own products, you reduce plastic waste and have more control over the ingredients in your home.

SUSTAINABLE HOUSEHOLD PRODUCTS

Castor oil-based cleaners support a more sustainable lifestyle, reducing the environmental impact associated with commercial cleaning products. The natural ingredients are biodegradable and can be safely disposed of without harming the ecosystem. Many of the remedies in this chapter are multi-functional, allowing you to use a single cleaner for multiple surfaces, further reducing waste and simplifying your cleaning routine.

Each of the following recipes is designed to maximize the cleaning power of castor oil while remaining environmentally friendly. These recipes provide effective, sustainable solutions for a variety of household cleaning needs, from removing stubborn stains to polishing furniture.

REMEDIES

Here are some eco-friendly home cleaning solutions featuring castor oil. Each remedy is crafted to be effective and safe for regular household use, combining castor oil with other natural ingredients to tackle common cleaning tasks.

116. All-Purpose Household Cleaner

Purpose: Cleans countertops, sinks, and other surfaces without leaving residue.

INGREDIENTS

- 1 tablespoon castor oil
- 1 cup distilled water
- 1/2 cup white vinegar
- 10 drops lemon essential oil

INSTRUCTIONS

1. Combine all ingredients in a spray bottle and shake well.
2. Spray onto surfaces and wipe with a cloth.

How to Use: Use as needed for general cleaning around the house.

117. Natural Castor Oil Soap

Purpose: A gentle, multi-purpose soap for hands, dishes, or surfaces.

INGREDIENTS

- 1/4 cup castor oil
- 1/4 cup coconut oil
- 1/2 cup liquid castile soap

INSTRUCTIONS

1. Melt coconut oil and combine with castor oil and castile soap.
2. Pour into a soap dispenser.

How to Use: Use as a hand soap, dish soap, or surface cleaner.

118. Castor Oil Furniture Polish

Purpose: Polishes and conditions wooden furniture, leaving a protective finish.

INGREDIENTS

- 1/4 cup castor oil
- 1/4 cup olive oil
- 5 drops lemon essential oil

INSTRUCTIONS

1. Mix all ingredients in a small bowl.
2. Apply a small amount to a cloth and rub onto wood surfaces.

How to Use: Buff with a clean cloth to a shine.

119. Pet-Safe Floor Cleaner

Purpose: Cleans floors without harmful chemicals, safe for homes with pets.

INGREDIENTS

- 1 tablespoon castor oil
- 1 gallon warm water
- 1/4 cup white vinegar

INSTRUCTIONS

1. Combine all ingredients in a bucket.
2. Use a mop or cloth to clean floors.

How to Use: Suitable for hardwood, tile, and vinyl floors.

120. Natural Dish Soap

Purpose: Cuts grease and cleans dishes without leaving chemical residues.

INGREDIENTS

- 2 tablespoons castor oil
- 1/2 cup liquid castile soap
- 10 drops lemon essential oil

INSTRUCTIONS

1. Mix ingredients in a bottle and shake.

How to Use: Use a few drops on a sponge for washing dishes.

121. Laundry Stain Remover

Purpose: Removes stains from clothing and fabrics naturally.

INGREDIENTS

- 1 tablespoon castor oil
- 1 tablespoon baking soda
- 1 tablespoon water

INSTRUCTIONS

1. Mix ingredients into a paste.
2. Apply to stains and let sit for 15 minutes before washing.

How to Use: Use as needed for stubborn stains.

122. Window and Glass Cleaner

Purpose: Leaves windows and mirrors streak-free and shiny.

INGREDIENTS

- 1 teaspoon castor oil
- 1 cup distilled water
- 1/2 cup white vinegar

INSTRUCTIONS

1. Combine ingredients in a spray bottle and shake well.
2. Spray onto glass surfaces and wipe with a microfiber cloth.

How to Use: Use as needed for glass and mirrors.

123. Castor Oil Mold and Mildew Remover

Purpose: Removes mold and mildew from bathroom tiles and grout.

INGREDIENTS

- 1 tablespoon castor oil
- 1/4 cup white vinegar
- 10 drops tea tree essential oil

INSTRUCTIONS

1. Mix all ingredients in a spray bottle.
2. Spray onto moldy areas and let sit for 15 minutes, then scrub.

How to Use: Use as needed in bathrooms or other damp areas.

124. Bathroom Scrub with Castor Oil

Purpose: Cleans bathroom surfaces, removing soap scum and grime.

INGREDIENTS

- 1 tablespoon castor oil
- 1/4 cup baking soda
- 1/4 cup white vinegar

INSTRUCTIONS

1. Combine baking soda and castor oil into a paste.
2. Add vinegar for a fizzing effect.

How to Use: Apply to surfaces, scrub, and rinse clean.

125. Toilet Bowl Cleaner

Purpose: Cleans and deodorizes the toilet bowl naturally.

INGREDIENTS

- 1 tablespoon castor oil
- 1/4 cup baking soda
- 10 drops eucalyptus essential oil

INSTRUCTIONS

1. Sprinkle baking soda in the toilet bowl.
2. Add castor oil and essential oil, scrub, and flush.

How to Use: Use weekly to maintain a fresh toilet bowl.

126. Oven and Grill Cleaner

Purpose: Removes grease and grime from ovens and grills.

INGREDIENTS

- 2 tablespoons castor oil
- 1/4 cup baking soda
- 1/4 cup vinegar

INSTRUCTIONS

1. Mix ingredients into a paste.
2. Apply to greasy areas and let sit for 20 minutes, then scrub.

How to Use: Rinse thoroughly after cleaning.

127. Carpet Stain Remover

Purpose: Lifts stains from carpets without harsh chemicals.

INGREDIENTS

- 1 tablespoon castor oil
- 1 tablespoon baking soda
- 1/4 cup water

INSTRUCTIONS

1. Mix ingredients into a paste.
2. Apply to stain, let sit for 15 minutes, then blot with a damp cloth.

How to Use: Use as needed for spot cleaning.

128. Silver Polish

Purpose: Cleans and polishes silverware and jewelry.

INGREDIENTS
- 1 tablespoon castor oil
- 1 tablespoon baking soda

INSTRUCTIONS
1. Combine ingredients into a paste.
2. Rub onto silver with a cloth, then rinse and buff.

How to Use: Use as needed for tarnished silver.

129. Kitchen Degreaser

Purpose: Cuts through grease on kitchen surfaces and appliances.

INGREDIENTS
- 1 tablespoon castor oil
- 1/2 cup white vinegar
- 10 drops lemon essential oil

INSTRUCTIONS
1. Mix all ingredients in a spray bottle.
2. Spray onto greasy surfaces and wipe clean.

How to Use: Ideal for stovetops, counters, and cabinets.

130. Castor Oil Room Spray

Purpose: Freshens the air without synthetic fragrances.

INGREDIENTS
- 1 tablespoon castor oil
- 1 cup distilled water
- 10 drops lavender essential oil (or preferred scent)

INSTRUCTIONS
1. Combine ingredients in a spray bottle and shake well.

How to Use: Spray around the room for a natural, fresh scent.

BOOK 10
PET CARE

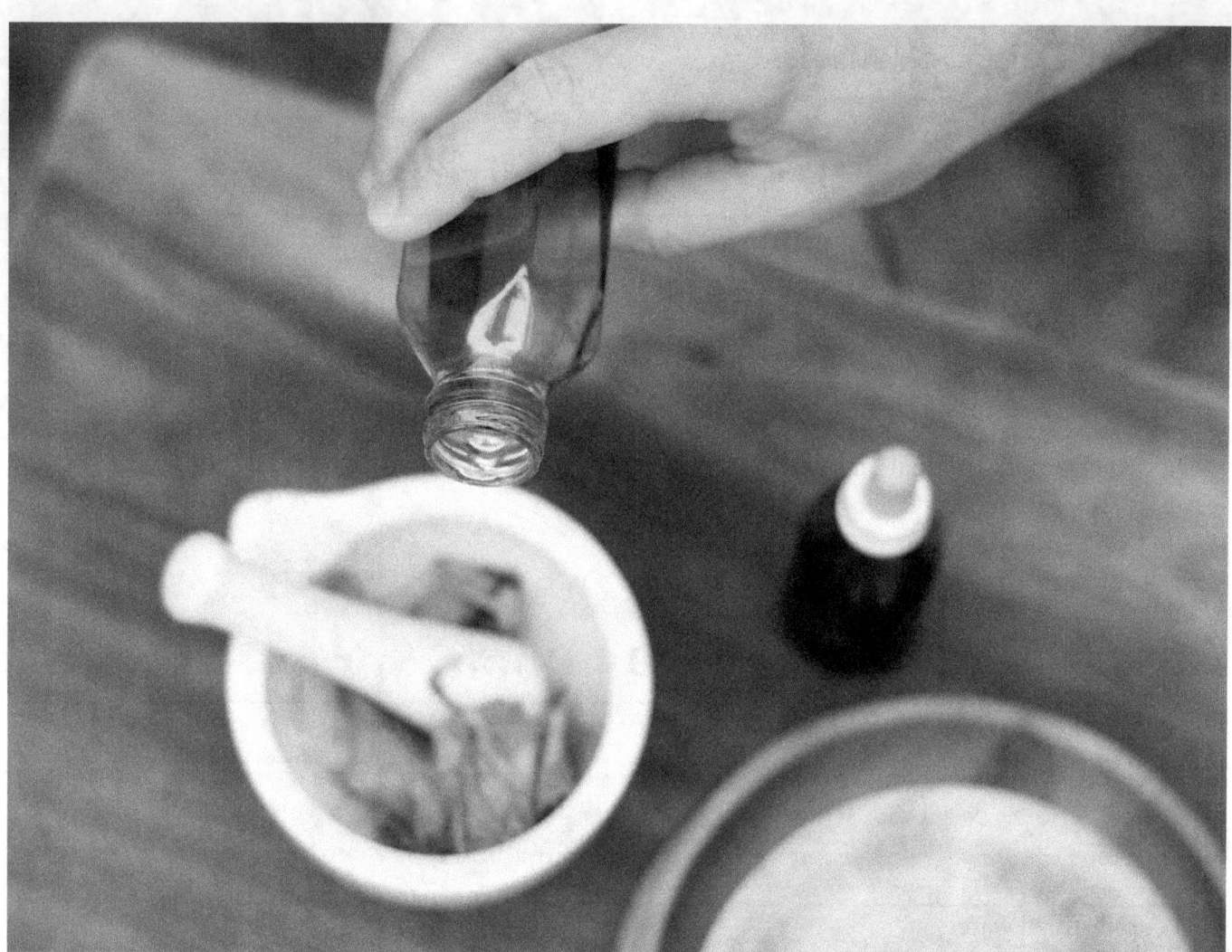

Caring for pets with natural remedies is becoming increasingly popular as more pet owners seek gentle, non-toxic solutions for common pet issues. Castor oil, with its anti-inflammatory, antimicrobial, and moisturizing properties, can be a helpful addition to your pet care routine. Whether it's for skin and coat health, flea prevention, or soothing irritations, castor oil provides a safe, effective alternative to many conventional pet care products. This chapter covers how castor oil can be used to maintain your pet's health and comfort, while also addressing common issues like itchy skin, hot spots, and minor wounds.

SKIN AND COAT CARE FOR PETS

Maintaining a healthy coat and skin is essential for a pet's well-being. Castor oil's natural emollient properties help moisturize dry skin, soothe irritations, and give the coat a soft, healthy shine. Castor oil can be used in shampoos, conditioning treatments, and leave-in serums to help keep a pet's coat looking its best. When combined with other natural ingredients, such as coconut oil or aloe vera, castor oil can effectively relieve dryness, reduce itchiness, and help prevent skin problems.

Regular grooming with castor oil-infused products can also reduce shedding and improve coat quality, making it easier to manage pet dander and maintain cleanliness around the home.

CASTOR OIL FOR PET HEALTH

Castor oil offers various benefits beyond skin care, providing natural support for issues like fleas, ticks, and ear health. When applied sparingly, castor oil can serve as a gentle flea repellent, keeping pests away without harsh chemicals. Its antimicrobial properties also make it an effective ear cleaner, helping prevent infections and maintain ear hygiene.

For pets with anxiety or restlessness, a castor oil-based massage can have a calming effect, promoting relaxation and improving circulation. Castor oil's versatility makes it a valuable tool for pet owners looking for holistic ways to care for their furry friends.

NATURAL FIRST AID FOR PETS

Minor cuts, scratches, and skin irritations are common in pets, especially those who spend time outdoors. Castor oil's antibacterial and antifungal properties make it ideal for treating minor wounds, soothing hot spots, and preventing infections. A small amount of castor oil applied to a cut or scratch can protect the area and promote faster healing.

For paw protection, castor oil can be used to create a balm that prevents paw pads from cracking due to rough surfaces or extreme temperatures. These remedies allow you to address common issues quickly and naturally, giving your pet the care they need without synthetic chemicals.

REMEDIES

Here are some castor oil remedies tailored specifically for pets, addressing common skin, coat, and health needs. Each remedy uses pet-safe ingredients to provide gentle yet effective care.

131. Pet Shampoo

Purpose: Cleanses and conditions pet's coat, leaving it soft and shiny.

INGREDIENTS

- 1 tablespoon castor oil
- 1/2 cup liquid castile soap
- 1 cup water
- 5 drops lavender essential oil (optional, for a calming scent)

INSTRUCTIONS

1. Combine all ingredients in a bottle and shake well.

How to Use: Apply to wet fur, lather gently, and rinse thoroughly.

132. Healing Balm for Paws and Skin

Purpose: Soothes cracked paws and dry skin, providing moisture and protection.

INGREDIENTS

- 1 tablespoon castor oil
- 1 tablespoon coconut oil
- 1 teaspoon beeswax

INSTRUCTIONS

1. Melt beeswax and coconut oil in a double boiler.
2. Add castor oil and stir well.
3. Pour into a small container and allow it to cool.

How to Use: Apply to paws and dry skin areas as needed.

133. Anti-Itch Remedy for Pets

Purpose: Relieves itching from allergies or dry skin.

INGREDIENTS

- 1 tablespoon castor oil
- 1 tablespoon aloe vera gel

INSTRUCTIONS

1. Mix castor oil and aloe vera gel in a small container.

How to Use: Apply to itchy areas, massaging gently into the skin.

134. Flea Prevention Rub

Purpose: Repels fleas naturally without harsh chemicals.

INGREDIENTS

- 1 tablespoon castor oil
- 1 tablespoon olive oil
- 5 drops eucalyptus essential oil (optional, for flea-repellent properties)

INSTRUCTIONS

1. Mix all ingredients in a small bottle.

How to Use: Rub a small amount on the back of the neck and base of the tail.

135. Ear Cleaning Solution

Purpose: Keeps ears clean and prevents infections.

INGREDIENTS

- 1 teaspoon castor oil
- 1 teaspoon olive oil

INSTRUCTIONS

1. Mix oils in a small dropper bottle.

How to Use: Apply a few drops to a cotton ball and gently wipe the inside of the ear.

136. Paw Pad Protector

Purpose: Protects paw pads from rough surfaces and extreme temperatures.

INGREDIENTS

- 1 tablespoon castor oil
- 1 tablespoon shea butter

INSTRUCTIONS

1. Melt shea butter and combine with castor oil.
2. Pour into a small container and let cool.

How to Use: Apply to paws before outdoor activities.

137. Hot Spot Relief Gel

Purpose: Relieves inflammation and itching from hot spots.

INGREDIENTS
- 1 tablespoon castor oil
- 1 tablespoon aloe vera gel

INSTRUCTIONS
1. Mix castor oil and aloe vera gel in a small container.

How to Use: Apply to affected areas 1-2 times daily.

138. Natural Anti-Tick Oil

Purpose: Helps repel ticks without chemicals.

INGREDIENTS
- 1 tablespoon castor oil
- 5 drops rosemary essential oil (optional)

INSTRUCTIONS
1. Mix oils in a small bottle.

How to Use: Apply a small amount to areas where ticks are likely, such as the neck or legs.

139. Pet Relaxation Massage Oil

Purpose: Promotes relaxation and reduces anxiety in pets.

INGREDIENTS
- 1 tablespoon castor oil
- 1 tablespoon almond oil
- 2 drops lavender essential oil (optional, for calming)

INSTRUCTIONS
1. Combine oils in a small bottle.

How to Use: Massage gently onto the back or neck for relaxation.

140. Pet Odor Remover

Purpose: Reduces pet odor naturally, leaving fur fresh.

INGREDIENTS

- 1 tablespoon castor oil
- 1/2 cup water
- 5 drops tea tree essential oil (optional, for odor control)

INSTRUCTIONS

1. Combine ingredients in a spray bottle and shake well.

How to Use: Lightly mist onto fur, avoiding the face, and wipe with a cloth.

141. Castor Oil for Pet Wounds

Purpose: Speeds healing and prevents infection in minor cuts.

INGREDIENTS

- 1 teaspoon castor oil

INSTRUCTIONS

1. Apply a small amount directly to the wound.

How to Use: Use daily until the wound heals.

142. Anti-Fungal Paw Spray

Purpose: Prevents fungal infections on paws, ideal for pets prone to yeast infections.

INGREDIENTS

- 1 tablespoon castor oil
- 1/2 cup water
- 5 drops tea tree essential oil (optional)

INSTRUCTIONS

1. Mix all ingredients in a spray bottle and shake.

How to Use: Spray onto paws and let air dry.

143. Castor Oil Ear Mite Treatment

Purpose: Helps remove ear mites and soothes irritation.

INGREDIENTS

- 1 teaspoon castor oil
- 1 drop neem oil (optional, for mite control)

INSTRUCTIONS

1. Combine oils in a small dropper bottle.

How to Use: Apply a few drops in the ear and gently massage the base.

144. Coat Shine Serum

Purpose: Adds shine and softness to pet fur.

INGREDIENTS

- 1 teaspoon castor oil
- 1 tablespoon coconut oil

INSTRUCTIONS

1. Mix oils in a small container.

How to Use: Rub a small amount onto the fur, avoiding the face.

145. Castor Oil for Pet Skin Allergies

Purpose: Soothes skin irritation from allergies and reduces inflammation.

INGREDIENTS

- 1 tablespoon castor oil
- 1 tablespoon chamomile tea (brewed and cooled)

INSTRUCTIONS

1. Mix chamomile tea and castor oil.

How to Use: Dab onto irritated areas with a cotton ball.

APPENDIX 1
RELAXATION AND WELLNESS

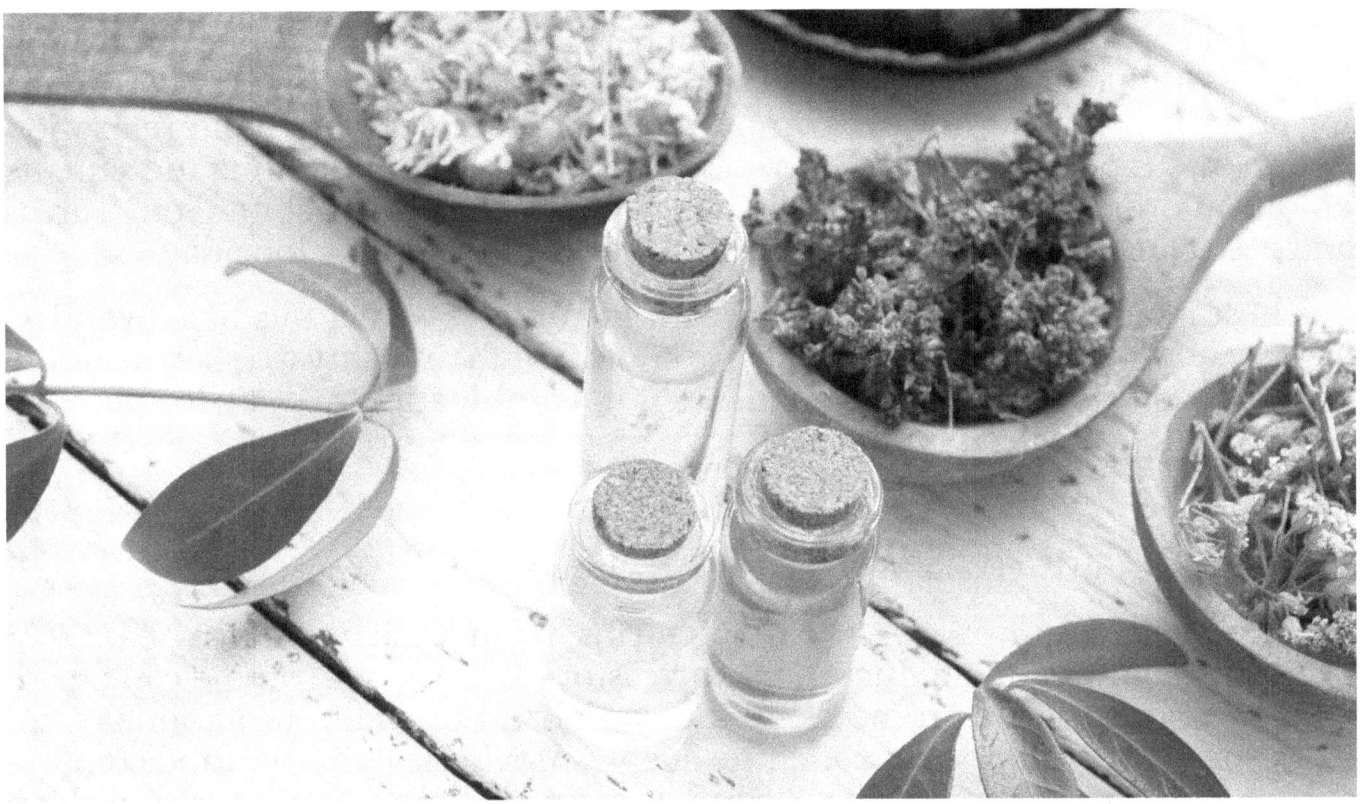

In today's fast-paced world, relaxation and wellness practices have become essential for mental and physical health. Castor oil, known for its moisturizing, soothing, and anti-inflammatory properties, can be an excellent addition to your relaxation routines. It can help reduce stress, promote restful sleep, and serve as a key ingredient in DIY wellness products, from massage oils to bath soaks. This chapter will explore how to incorporate castor oil into self-care practices to create a calming, rejuvenating environment.

CASTOR OIL FOR RELAXATION

Castor oil's gentle, penetrating warmth can soothe muscles, calm the mind, and hydrate the skin, making it a natural choice for relaxation. When combined with essential oils such as lavender or chamomile, castor oil creates a deeply relaxing experience, perfect for bedtime or moments of stress. Its viscosity also makes it ideal for massage oils, providing a smooth, gliding texture that relaxes the body while moisturizing the skin.

Using castor oil in relaxation practices can be as simple as adding a few drops to a warm bath or massaging it onto pressure points. It's an effective way to create a moment of tranquility and bring balance to your daily routine.

STRESS RELIEF APPLICATIONS

Stress relief is a critical part of self-care, and castor oil offers a versatile foundation for stress-reducing remedies. Whether used in an aromatherapy blend, a soothing foot soak, or a calming eye compress, castor oil can enhance your relaxation efforts by supporting circulation, reducing tension, and nourishing the skin. Its emollient properties make it especially comforting, helping to soften rough areas and ease sore muscles, which is perfect for unwinding after a long day.

For best results, combine castor oil with calming essential oils like lavender, ylang-ylang, or bergamot. These oils are known for their ability to relax the mind, reduce anxiety, and improve mood. Used in combination with castor oil, they offer a gentle yet effective approach to managing daily stress.

SELF-CARE PRACTICES WITH CASTOR OIL

Self-care with castor oil can take many forms, from a warm, relaxing bath to a soothing hand treatment. Incorporating castor oil into your routine can create a nurturing ritual that promotes both physical and mental relaxation. Its rich, thick consistency allows it to penetrate deeply, providing hydration and comfort that lasts. Castor oil can also be used in homemade balms, body oils, and sleep aids, providing a natural alternative to synthetic products.

The following remedies are designed to help you unwind, relieve tension, and indulge in moments of peace. With simple ingredients and easy-to-follow steps, you can transform your self-care routine into a calming, spa-like experience at home.

REMEDIES

Here are some relaxing and wellness-focused remedies featuring castor oil. Each remedy has been crafted to provide comfort, relieve stress, and enhance relaxation through simple, natural ingredients.

146. Relaxing Bath Soak with Castor Oil and Essential Oils

Purpose: Relieves tension and relaxes muscles, creating a spa-like bath experience.

INGREDIENTS

- 2 tablespoons castor oil
- 1/2 cup Epsom salts
- 10 drops lavender essential oil

INSTRUCTIONS

1. Mix castor oil and lavender essential oil.
2. Sprinkle Epsom salts and castor oil blend into a warm bath.

How to Use: Soak for 20-30 minutes, breathing deeply to relax.

147. Castor Oil Aromatherapy Blend

Purpose: Calms the mind and uplifts mood through aromatherapy.

INGREDIENTS

- 1 tablespoon castor oil
- 5 drops bergamot essential oil
- 3 drops ylang-ylang essential oil

INSTRUCTIONS

1. Combine all ingredients in a small bottle.
2. Shake well to mix.

How to Use: Dab onto wrists or inhale directly for an uplifting scent.

148. Calming Massage Oil

Purpose: Relieves muscle tension and promotes relaxation.

INGREDIENTS

- 2 tablespoons castor oil
- 1 tablespoon almond oil
- 5 drops chamomile essential oil

INSTRUCTIONS

1. Mix all ingredients in a small bottle.
2. Shake well before use.

How to Use: Massage into tense muscles or use as a full-body relaxation oil.

149. Foot Soak for Stress Relief

Purpose: Eases foot tension and promotes relaxation.

INGREDIENTS

- 1 tablespoon castor oil
- 1/4 cup Epsom salts
- 5 drops peppermint essential oil (optional)

INSTRUCTIONS

1. Fill a basin with warm water, adding castor oil, Epsom salts, and essential oil.

How to Use: Soak feet for 15-20 minutes, then pat dry.

150. Castor Oil Lavender Eye Compress

Purpose: Reduces puffiness and relieves eye strain.

INGREDIENTS

- 1 tablespoon castor oil
- 3 drops lavender essential oil
- Soft cloth

INSTRUCTIONS

1. Mix castor oil and lavender oil.
2. Soak the cloth in the oil blend, then place over closed eyes.

How to Use: Relax with the compress over your eyes for 10 minutes.

151. DIY Sleep Aid Balm

Purpose: Promotes restful sleep and relaxation.

INGREDIENTS

- 1 tablespoon castor oil
- 1 tablespoon coconut oil
- 5 drops lavender essential oil

INSTRUCTIONS

1. Combine all ingredients in a small jar.
2. Stir well until blended.

How to Use: Apply to wrists and temples before bedtime.

152. Castor Oil Meditation Balm

Purpose: Enhances meditation by calming the mind and relaxing the body.

INGREDIENTS
- 1 tablespoon castor oil
- 5 drops sandalwood essential oil

INSTRUCTIONS
1. Mix oils in a small container.

How to Use: Apply to temples and wrists before meditating.

153. Castor Oil Head Massage for Relaxation

Purpose: Relieves tension and soothes the scalp for relaxation.

INGREDIENTS
- 2 tablespoons castor oil
- 1 tablespoon coconut oil

INSTRUCTIONS
1. Combine oils and mix well.

How to Use: Massage onto scalp and let sit for 15-20 minutes before rinsing.

154. Anti-Anxiety Body Balm

Purpose: Reduces anxiety and promotes relaxation through touch.

INGREDIENTS
- 1 tablespoon castor oil
- 1 tablespoon shea butter
- 5 drops frankincense essential oil

INSTRUCTIONS
1. Melt shea butter and mix with castor oil and essential oil.
2. Pour into a small jar to cool.

How to Use: Massage onto chest and shoulders for a calming effect.

155. Stress-Reducing Body Oil

Purpose: Eases stress and hydrates the skin, perfect for evening relaxation.

INGREDIENTS

- 2 tablespoons castor oil
- 1 tablespoon jojoba oil
- 5 drops clary sage essential oil

INSTRUCTIONS

1. Combine ingredients in a small bottle and shake well.

How to Use: Massage onto the body, especially the neck and shoulders.

156. Mood-Boosting Roller Blend

Purpose: Uplifts mood and reduces stress.

INGREDIENTS

- 1 tablespoon castor oil
- 5 drops orange essential oil
- 3 drops geranium essential oil

INSTRUCTIONS

1. Mix ingredients in a roller bottle and shake.

How to Use: Apply to wrists and inhale as needed.

157. Peaceful Sleep Pillow Spray

Purpose: Encourages restful sleep with a calming scent.

INGREDIENTS

- 1/2 teaspoon castor oil
- 1 cup distilled water
- 10 drops lavender essential oil

INSTRUCTIONS

1. Combine ingredients in a spray bottle and shake well.

How to Use: Mist onto your pillow and bedding before sleep.

158. Hand and Nail Moisturizing Treatment

Purpose: Soothes and hydrates hands, promoting nail health.

INGREDIENTS

- 1 tablespoon castor oil
- 1 tablespoon olive oil
- 3 drops lavender essential oil

INSTRUCTIONS

1. Mix oils in a small bowl.

How to Use: Massage into hands and nails, then let sit for 10 minutes before rinsing.

159. DIY Candle with Castor Oil

Purpose: Creates a relaxing atmosphere with a subtle, natural scent.

INGREDIENTS

- 1/4 cup castor oil
- 1/2 cup beeswax
- 10 drops lavender essential oil
- Wick and container

INSTRUCTIONS

1. Melt beeswax and castor oil together, then add essential oil.
2. Pour into the container with the wick and let cool.

How to Use: Light the candle to enhance relaxation.

160. Castor Oil Relaxation Candle

Purpose: Provides calming ambiance and releases a gentle aroma.

INGREDIENTS

- 1/4 cup castor oil
- 1/2 cup soy wax
- 10 drops chamomile essential oil

INSTRUCTIONS

1. Melt soy wax and mix in castor oil and chamomile oil.
2. Pour into a candle holder with a wick.

How to Use: Light to create a peaceful atmosphere.

APPENDIX 2
INSIGHTS FROM DR. BARBARA'S RESEARCH

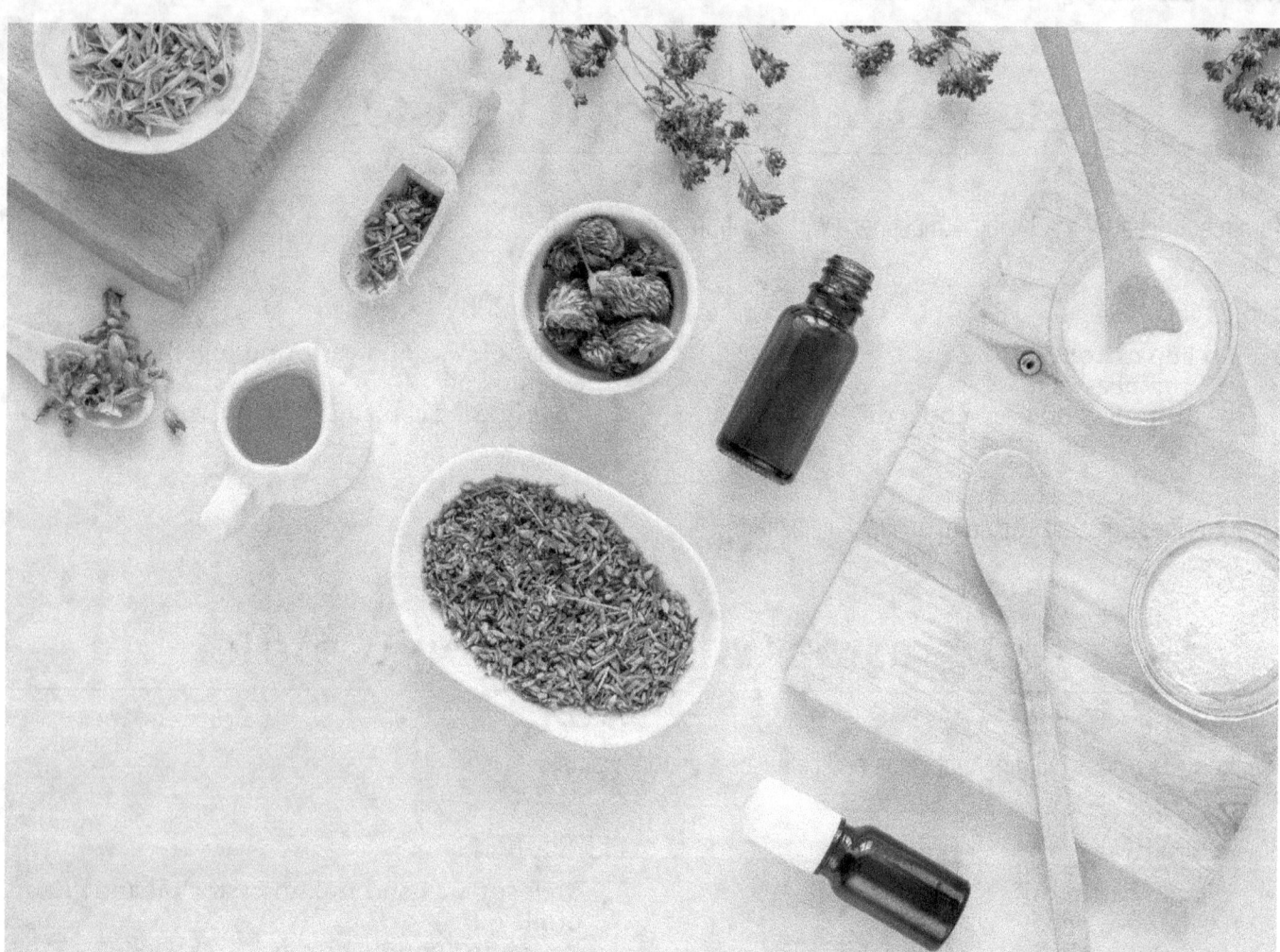

Dr. Barbara's research into the healing properties of castor oil highlights its potential as a versatile, natural remedy for a variety of health and wellness applications. Through years of scientific study and practical experience, Dr. Barbara has explored how castor oil can support physical, mental, and emotional well-being. In this chapter, we'll delve into the scientific research behind castor oil, share transformative stories from individuals who have experienced its benefits, and explore integrative approaches to using castor oil for mind-body wellness. This section also includes remedies designed to support holistic health, integrating both traditional and modern insights into castor oil's uses.

SCIENTIFIC RESEARCH ON CASTOR OIL'S BENEFITS

Dr. Barbara's research has uncovered a wealth of information on castor oil's medicinal properties, particularly its anti-inflammatory, antimicrobial, and immune-supporting effects. The primary component of castor oil, ricinoleic acid, has been shown in studies to reduce inflammation and relieve pain when applied topically. This effect is due to ricinoleic acid's ability to inhibit certain molecules responsible for pain and inflammation, which makes castor oil effective in treating conditions such as arthritis, muscle soreness, and joint discomfort.

Additionally, castor oil's unique composition allows it to penetrate deeply into the skin, providing targeted relief to tissues and improving circulation. Studies have shown that applying castor oil packs to the abdomen can support lymphatic drainage and detoxification, promoting liver health and aiding in the body's natural elimination processes. Dr. Barbara's research emphasizes the importance of using castor oil in its purest form, as unrefined castor oil retains more of its natural therapeutic properties.

REAL-LIFE TRANSFORMATIONS WITH CASTOR OIL

Dr. Barbara's clients and research participants have reported remarkable transformations using castor oil for a variety of health concerns. From chronic pain relief to improved skin health, these stories illustrate castor oil's potential as a natural remedy. For instance, individuals with arthritis have experienced reduced joint stiffness and pain after consistent use of castor oil packs. Athletes and active individuals have noted faster recovery times and less muscle soreness with castor oil massage and post-exercise balms.

One particularly inspiring case involved a woman who used castor oil to manage symptoms of anxiety and insomnia. By incorporating castor oil into her nightly routine—through a calming massage oil and a sleep support pack—she experienced greater relaxation and improved sleep quality. These real-life transformations reinforce Dr. Barbara's belief in castor oil's holistic benefits, extending beyond physical health to support mental and emotional well-being.

INTEGRATIVE APPROACHES

Dr. Barbara advocates for an integrative approach to wellness that combines castor oil with other healing modalities, such as aromatherapy, reflexology, and energy work. Castor oil's compatibility with essential oils and its effectiveness in various types of massage make it ideal for integrative practices. For instance, using castor oil in reflexology massages can stimulate key pressure points, enhancing energy flow throughout the body. Dr. Barbara also recommends pairing castor oil with meditation or chakra alignment practices, as its soothing properties support a calm, focused mind.

Integrating castor oil into wellness routines aligns with Dr. Barbara's philosophy of addressing both body and mind for comprehensive health benefits. Whether used as part of a detox protocol, in massage therapy, or in energy-balancing routines, castor oil offers a unique and flexible approach to self-care.

REMEDIES

The following remedies blend Dr. Barbara's research findings with practical applications, offering ways to incorporate castor oil into holistic wellness practices. These remedies are designed to support both physical and emotional health, providing tools for relaxation, energy balance, and enhanced recovery.

161. Mind-Body Wellness Oil

Purpose: Supports mental clarity and physical relaxation through aromatherapy.

INGREDIENTS
- 1 tablespoon castor oil
- 5 drops frankincense essential oil
- 3 drops lavender essential oil

INSTRUCTIONS
1. Mix all ingredients in a small bottle.
2. Shake well to blend.

How to Use: Apply to pulse points or use in meditation for calming effects.

162. Energy Balancing Body Balm

Purpose: Enhances energy flow and provides grounding, especially useful during meditation.

INGREDIENTS
- 1 tablespoon castor oil
- 1 tablespoon shea butter
- 3 drops sandalwood essential oil

INSTRUCTIONS
1. Melt shea butter, then mix with castor oil and essential oil.
2. Pour into a small container and let cool.

How to Use: Massage onto hands, wrists, and chest for grounding energy.

163. Chakra Aligning Oil Blend

Purpose: Supports chakra alignment and energy flow through gentle massage.

INGREDIENTS

- 1 tablespoon castor oil
- 1 drop each of rose, jasmine, and ylang-ylang essential oils

INSTRUCTIONS

1. Mix all ingredients in a small bottle.

How to Use: Apply to chakra points during meditation or energy work.

164. Immune-Boosting Castor Oil

Purpose: Enhances immune function through application to lymph nodes.

INGREDIENTS

- 1 tablespoon castor oil
- 3 drops tea tree essential oil (antibacterial)

INSTRUCTIONS

1. Mix castor oil and tea tree oil in a small bottle.

How to Use: Apply to lymph areas (neck, underarms) once weekly.

165. Deep Tissue Relief Oil

Purpose: Relieves muscle soreness and supports deep tissue recovery.

INGREDIENTS

- 1 tablespoon castor oil
- 1 tablespoon arnica oil
- 5 drops eucalyptus essential oil

INSTRUCTIONS

1. Combine all ingredients in a small container.

How to Use: Massage into sore muscles or joints after exercise.

166. Detoxifying Foot Balm

Purpose: Supports detoxification through foot application.

INGREDIENTS

- 1 tablespoon castor oil
- 1 tablespoon coconut oil
- 5 drops peppermint essential oil

INSTRUCTIONS

1. Mix ingredients and pour into a small jar.

How to Use: Massage onto feet before bed for detox benefits.

167. Reflexology Massage Oil

Purpose: Enhances reflexology sessions by supporting energy flow and circulation.

INGREDIENTS

- 1 tablespoon castor oil
- 1 tablespoon olive oil

INSTRUCTIONS

1. Combine oils and stir well.

How to Use: Use on feet and hands during reflexology massage.

168. Post-Exercise Recovery Balm

Purpose: Reduces muscle stiffness and speeds recovery after workouts.

INGREDIENTS

- 1 tablespoon castor oil
- 1 tablespoon shea butter
- 5 drops rosemary essential oil

INSTRUCTIONS

1. Melt shea butter and combine with castor oil and rosemary oil.
2. Pour into a container and let cool.

How to Use: Apply to sore muscles and let absorb.

169. Circulation Enhancing Balm

Purpose: Improves circulation and reduces tension in the legs and feet.

INGREDIENTS

- 1 tablespoon castor oil
- 1 tablespoon coconut oil
- 5 drops ginger essential oil

INSTRUCTIONS

1. Mix all ingredients in a small jar.

How to Use: Massage into legs and feet for circulation support.

170. Sleep Support Castor Pack

Purpose: Promotes restful sleep by relaxing the body and mind.

INGREDIENTS

- 1 tablespoon castor oil
- Cotton cloth
- Heating pad

INSTRUCTIONS

1. Soak the cloth in castor oil and wring out excess.
2. Place on abdomen and cover with a heating pad for 15-20 minutes.

How to Use: Use before bedtime to encourage relaxation and sleep.

APPENDIX 3
DIY – CRAFTING CASTOR OIL PREPARATIONS

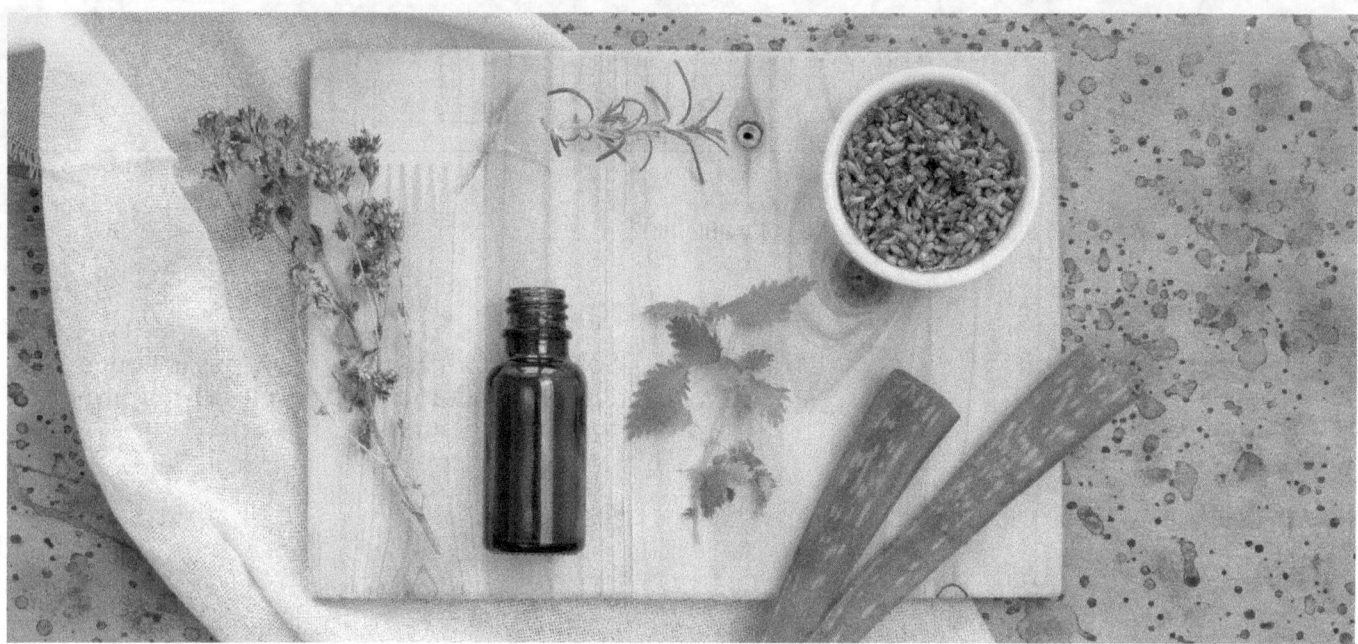

Creating your own castor oil-based products at home allows you to tailor natural remedies to your specific needs. From tinctures and infused oils to lotions and balms, castor oil can be combined with various ingredients to create personalized products that are both effective and nourishing. This chapter will guide you through the basics of DIY castor oil preparations, offering tips, instructions, and easy-to-follow recipes to craft your own lotions, serums, and more. By using simple ingredients and techniques, you can enjoy the full benefits of castor oil in its purest form, free from synthetic additives.

CREATING HERBAL TINCTURES AND INFUSED OILS

Infusing castor oil with herbs is a powerful way to enhance its healing properties. Herbs like calendula, lavender, and chamomile can add extra anti-inflammatory, antimicrobial, and soothing effects, making the infused oil even more versatile.

Herbal tinctures and infusions are easy to make at home and can be used in a variety of ways—from soothing irritated skin to easing muscle pain.

To create an infused oil, combine dried herbs with castor oil in a glass jar, seal tightly, and let it steep in a warm place for 2-4 weeks. Strain the oil to remove the herbs, and you'll have a potent, herbal-infused castor oil ready for use.

INSTRUCTIONS AND TIPS FOR DIY PREPARATIONS

Making your own castor oil products at home is simple, but there are a few tips to ensure success:

Choose Quality Ingredients: Use organic, unrefined castor oil and fresh herbs or high-quality essential oils to maintain purity and potency.

Sanitize Containers: Clean and sanitize jars and containers before use to prevent contamination.

Store Properly: Keep DIY products in dark, glass containers to extend shelf life and prevent oxidation. Store them in a cool, dry place.

With these basics in mind, you'll be ready to craft personalized castor oil products tailored to your wellness needs.

PERSONALIZED CASTOR OIL PRODUCTS

Personalizing your castor oil preparations allows you to address specific skin, hair, or health concerns. Whether you're making a moisturizing lotion, an anti-itch spray, or a soothing body butter, you can adjust the ingredients and essential oils to match your preferences. These custom-made products make wonderful gifts or additions to your own wellness routine.

LOTIONS, SERUMS, AND OINTMENTS

Castor oil is an excellent base for creating skin-nourishing products like lotions, serums, and ointments. Its thick consistency and moisturizing properties make it ideal for dry or irritated skin, while its anti-inflammatory benefits provide relief from conditions like eczema or sunburn. By combining castor oil with other nourishing ingredients like shea butter, vitamin E, and essential oils, you can create a range of effective products for different skin needs.

REMEDIES

Here are DIY recipes for castor oil-based products, covering everything from herbal infusions to body lotions and balms. These preparations offer a simple, natural approach to skin care, wellness, and personal care.

171. Castor Oil Infused Herbal Tincture

Purpose: Enhances the healing properties of castor oil by infusing it with herbs.

INGREDIENTS

- 1 cup castor oil
- 1/4 cup dried calendula or chamomile flowers

INSTRUCTIONS

1. Place herbs in a glass jar and cover with castor oil.
2. Seal and let infuse in a warm place for 2-4 weeks.
3. Strain out herbs and store the oil.

How to Use: Apply to skin for soothing and anti-inflammatory benefits.

172. Soothing Moisturizing Lotion

Purpose: Hydrates and soothes dry skin, leaving it soft and supple.

INGREDIENTS

- 1/4 cup castor oil
- 1/4 cup aloe vera gel
- 1/4 cup coconut oil

INSTRUCTIONS

1. Melt coconut oil and mix with castor oil and aloe vera gel.
2. Stir until well combined and pour into a container.

How to Use: Apply to dry skin as needed.

173. Natural Sunscreen with Castor Oil

Purpose: Provides light sun protection and moisturizes skin.

INGREDIENTS

- 1/4 cup castor oil
- 1/4 cup shea butter
- 1 tablespoon zinc oxide

INSTRUCTIONS

1. Melt shea butter, add castor oil and zinc oxide, and mix well.

How to Use: Apply to skin before sun exposure.

174. Vitamin E Infused Body Oil

Purpose: Nourishes skin and provides antioxidant protection.

INGREDIENTS
- 1/4 cup castor oil
- 1 tablespoon vitamin E oil

INSTRUCTIONS
1. Mix castor oil and vitamin E in a small bottle.

How to Use: Massage onto skin after a shower for hydration.

175. Castor Oil Roll-On Pain Reliever

Purpose: Provides targeted relief for sore muscles and joints.

INGREDIENTS
- 1 tablespoon castor oil
- 5 drops peppermint essential oil
- Roll-on bottle

INSTRUCTIONS
1. Combine ingredients and pour into a roll-on bottle.

How to Use: Apply to sore areas as needed.

176. DIY Anti-Itch Spray

Purpose: Relieves itching from insect bites or skin irritations.

INGREDIENTS
- 1/4 cup castor oil
- 1/4 cup distilled water
- 5 drops tea tree essential oil

INSTRUCTIONS
1. Mix all ingredients in a spray bottle and shake.

How to Use: Spray onto itchy areas for relief.

177. Natural Lip Balm with Castor Oil

Purpose: Keeps lips hydrated and smooth.

INGREDIENTS

- 1 tablespoon castor oil
- 1 tablespoon beeswax

INSTRUCTIONS

1. Melt beeswax and mix with castor oil.
2. Pour into a lip balm container and let cool.

How to Use: Apply to lips as needed.

178. Cuticle Oil for Nail Health

Purpose: Nourishes cuticles and strengthens nails.

INGREDIENTS

- 1 tablespoon castor oil
- 1 tablespoon jojoba oil

INSTRUCTIONS

1. Mix oils in a small bottle.

How to Use: Massage into cuticles daily.

179. Castor Oil and Calendula Healing Salve

Purpose: Heals minor cuts and soothes irritated skin.

INGREDIENTS

- 1/4 cup castor oil
- 1/4 cup dried calendula flowers
- 1 tablespoon beeswax

INSTRUCTIONS

1. Infuse castor oil with calendula (as above).
2. Melt beeswax, add infused oil, and stir.

How to Use: Apply to minor cuts or scrapes.

180. DIY Perfume Balm with Castor Oil

Purpose: Provides a subtle scent with moisturizing benefits.

INGREDIENTS

- 1 tablespoon castor oil
- 1 tablespoon beeswax
- 10 drops essential oil (your preferred scent)

INSTRUCTIONS

1. Melt beeswax and mix with castor oil and essential oil.
2. Pour into a small container and let cool.

How to Use: Dab onto pulse points.

181. Deep Moisturizing Hand Cream

Purpose: Keeps hands soft and prevents dryness.

INGREDIENTS

- 1/4 cup castor oil
- 1/4 cup shea butter

INSTRUCTIONS

1. Melt shea butter and mix with castor oil.

How to Use: Apply to hands as needed.

182. Castor Oil Foot Scrub

Purpose: Exfoliates and softens rough feet.

INGREDIENTS

- 1/4 cup castor oil
- 1/4 cup sugar

INSTRUCTIONS

1. Mix ingredients into a paste.

How to Use: Massage onto feet and rinse.

183. Smoothing Body Butter

Purpose: Provides deep moisture for dry skin.

INGREDIENTS

- 1/4 cup castor oil
- 1/4 cup cocoa butter

INSTRUCTIONS

1. Melt cocoa butter and mix with castor oil.

How to Use: Massage onto skin for hydration.

184. Aloe and Castor After-Sun Lotion

Purpose: Soothes sun-exposed skin.

INGREDIENTS

- 1/4 cup castor oil
- 1/4 cup aloe vera gel

INSTRUCTIONS

1. Mix ingredients in a small bottle.

How to Use: Apply to sun-exposed skin.

185. DIY Hand Sanitizer with Castor Oil

Purpose: Cleans hands while moisturizing.

INGREDIENTS

- 1 tablespoon castor oil
- 1/2 cup rubbing alcohol
- 10 drops tea tree essential oil

INSTRUCTIONS

1. Mix all ingredients in a spray bottle.

How to Use: Spray on hands and rub together.

186. Insect Repellent Balm

Purpose: Repels insects naturally.

INGREDIENTS
- 1/4 cup castor oil
- 10 drops citronella essential oil

INSTRUCTIONS
1. Mix ingredients in a container.

How to Use: Apply to exposed skin.

187. Herbal Infusion Oil

Purpose: Versatile base for other DIY products.

INGREDIENTS
- 1 cup castor oil
- 1/4 cup dried lavender

INSTRUCTIONS
1. Infuse as directed above.

How to Use: Use as a base for lotions and balms.

188. Castor Oil Solid Perfume

Purpose: Subtle fragrance in solid form.

INGREDIENTS
- 1 tablespoon castor oil
- 1 tablespoon beeswax
- 10 drops essential oil

INSTRUCTIONS
1. Melt beeswax, add oils, pour into a small tin.

189. Castor Oil-Based Deodorant

Purpose: Provides a natural alternative to commercial deodorants, offering odor control and skin hydration.

INGREDIENTS

- 1 tablespoon castor oil
- 1 tablespoon coconut oil
- 1 tablespoon baking soda
- 5 drops tea tree essential oil

INSTRUCTIONS

- Melt coconut oil and mix with castor oil.
- Add baking soda and essential oil, stirring well.
- Pour into a small container and let cool.

How to Use: Apply a small amount under the arms for freshness.

190. Hair Shine Serum

Purpose: Adds shine and softness to hair, taming frizz and smoothing ends.

INGREDIENTS

- 1 tablespoon castor oil
- 1 tablespoon argan oil

INSTRUCTIONS

1. Combine oils in a small bottle and shake well.

How to Use: Apply a few drops to the ends of damp or dry hair.

191. Relaxing Massage Balm

Purpose: Eases muscle tension and promotes relaxation through massage.

INGREDIENTS

- 1 tablespoon castor oil
- 1 tablespoon shea butter
- 5 drops lavender essential oil

INSTRUCTIONS

1. Melt shea butter, then mix in castor oil and lavender oil.
2. Pour into a small jar and let cool.

How to Use: Massage onto tense areas to soothe muscles.

192. Cleansing Oil for Face

Purpose: Gently cleanses the skin, removing impurities and makeup.

INGREDIENTS
- 1 tablespoon castor oil
- 1 tablespoon jojoba oil

INSTRUCTIONS
1. Mix oils in a small bottle and shake.

How to Use: Massage onto face, then wipe off with a warm, damp cloth.

193. DIY Makeup Remover Wipes

Purpose: Removes makeup gently, leaving skin clean and hydrated.

INGREDIENTS
- 1 tablespoon castor oil
- 1/2 cup distilled water
- Cotton pads

INSTRUCTIONS
1. Mix castor oil and water in a small bowl.
2. Soak cotton pads in the mixture and store in a jar.

How to Use: Wipe gently over face to remove makeup.

194. Calming Chest Rub

Purpose: Provides soothing relief and supports respiratory health.

INGREDIENTS
- 1 tablespoon castor oil
- 5 drops eucalyptus essential oil

INSTRUCTIONS
1. Mix castor oil and eucalyptus oil in a small jar.

How to Use: Rub onto the chest and neck for calming effects.

195. Cooling Relief Gel

Purpose: Soothes skin irritation and provides a cooling effect.

INGREDIENTS

- 1 tablespoon castor oil
- 1/4 cup aloe vera gel
- 5 drops peppermint essential oil

INSTRUCTIONS

1. Mix ingredients in a container until smooth.

How to Use: Apply to irritated skin for cooling relief.

196. Foot Hydrating Mask

Purpose: Deeply moisturizes and softens rough feet.

INGREDIENTS

- 1 tablespoon castor oil
- 1 tablespoon honey

INSTRUCTIONS

1. Combine castor oil and honey in a small bowl.

How to Use: Apply to feet, cover with socks, and leave on for 20 minutes before rinsing.

197. Castor Oil Hair Detangler

Purpose: Eases tangles and smooths hair, making it easier to manage.

INGREDIENTS

- 1 tablespoon castor oil
- 1/2 cup distilled water
- 5 drops lavender essential oil

INSTRUCTIONS

1. Mix ingredients in a spray bottle and shake well.

How to Use: Spray onto damp hair and comb through.

198. Natural Bug Bite Soother

Purpose: Relieves itching and discomfort from bug bites.

INGREDIENTS
- 1 teaspoon castor oil
- 1 teaspoon aloe vera gel

INSTRUCTIONS
1. Mix ingredients in a small container.

How to Use: Apply to bug bites as needed for relief.

199. Castor Oil Stretch Mark Cream

Purpose: Reduces the appearance of stretch marks and improves skin elasticity.

INGREDIENTS
- 1 tablespoon castor oil
- 1 tablespoon cocoa butter
- 5 drops vitamin E oil

INSTRUCTIONS
1. Melt cocoa butter and mix with castor oil and vitamin E.

How to Use: Massage onto areas with stretch marks daily.

200. Castor Oil Tincture for Immune Health

Purpose: Supports immune function through a topical application.

INGREDIENTS
- 1 tablespoon castor oil
- 1 tablespoon olive oil
- 5 drops oregano essential oil

INSTRUCTIONS
1. Mix ingredients in a small bottle.

How to Use: Massage onto chest or neck as part of a wellness routine.

201. Herbal Healing Oil for Skin Rejuvenation

Purpose: Promotes skin renewal and rejuvenates dull or damaged skin.

INGREDIENTS
- 1/4 cup castor oil
- 1/4 cup dried lavender or chamomile flowers

INSTRUCTIONS
1. Infuse castor oil with dried flowers for 2-4 weeks, then strain.

How to Use: Apply to face and neck nightly for rejuvenating effects.

APPENDIX 4
EMOTIONAL BALANCE AND MENTAL CLARITY

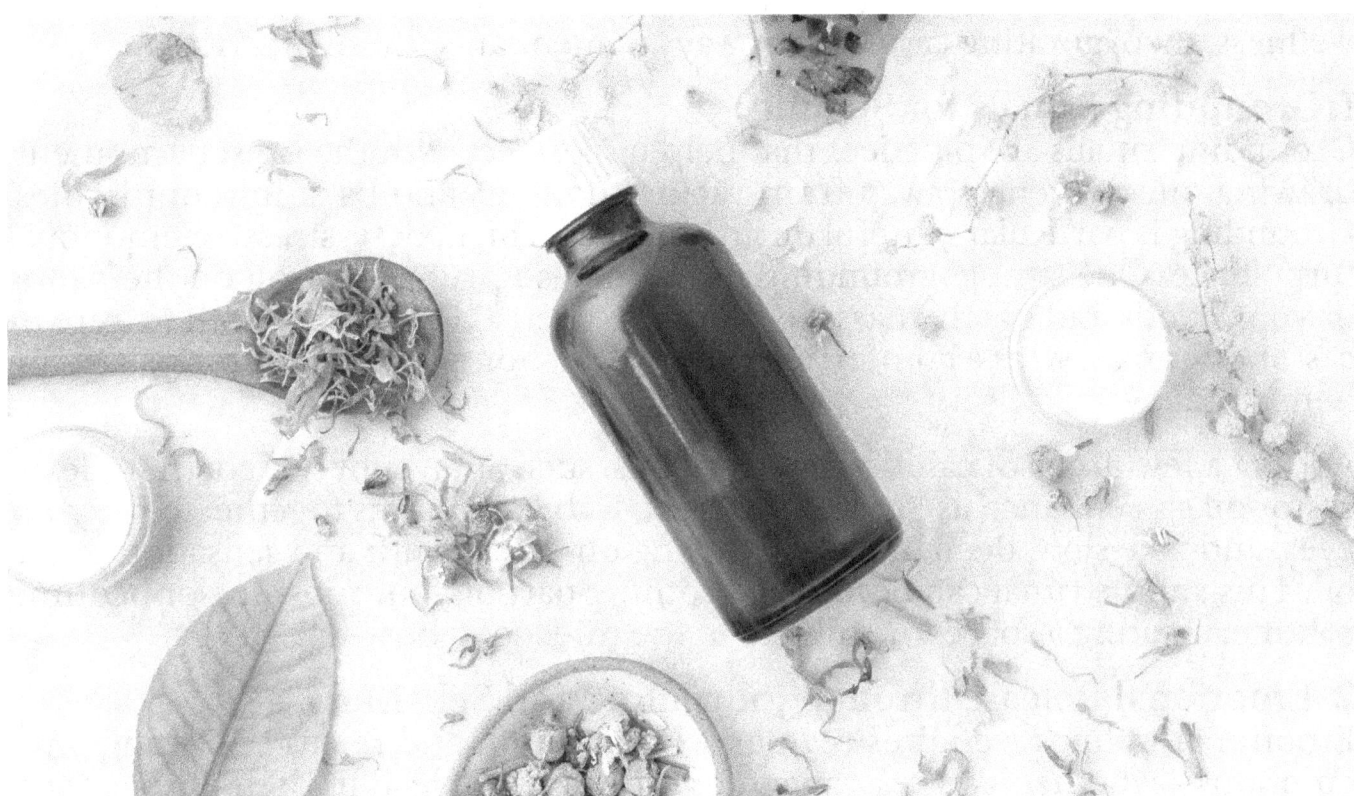

In today's fast-paced world, finding emotional balance and maintaining mental clarity can feel like constant challenges. Between work obligations, family responsibilities, and the demands of modern life, it's easy to feel overwhelmed, anxious, and distracted. However, achieving a state of emotional calm and mental focus is essential for leading a fulfilling and healthy life. This chapter explores practical techniques for cultivating emotional wellness and enhancing mental clarity, and how castor oil, known for its physical healing properties, can be integrated into routines that support a calm mind and balanced emotions.

Emotional balance and mental clarity are not about eliminating stress or achieving perfection. Instead, they involve building resilience, developing self-awareness, and nurturing the ability to stay present and focused, even when faced with challenges. Castor oil, when combined with mindful techniques and natural wellness practices, can serve as a valuable tool in this journey. Its soothing properties, grounding texture, and compatibility with essential oils make it a perfect addition to routines designed to support emotional and mental well-being.

TECHNIQUES FOR EMOTIONAL WELLNESS

Emotional wellness is the foundation of mental health. It involves understanding our emotions, developing strategies to manage stress, and cultivating practices that foster calm and inner peace. When we are emotionally balanced, we are better able to handle life's ups and downs, connect meaningfully with others, and stay grounded in our values. Here are some techniques for nurturing emotional wellness, incorporating castor oil in ways that enhance these practices.

1. Grounding Rituals for Stability

Grounding rituals are practices that help us connect with the present moment, drawing our awareness away from racing thoughts and back into our bodies. Grounding is particularly useful during moments of anxiety, stress, or emotional turbulence. One simple grounding technique is to rub castor oil on the palms of your hands and gently massage them together. The thick, smooth texture of castor oil can serve as a comforting physical anchor, pulling your focus into the here and now.

Adding a few drops of calming essential oils, such as lavender or chamomile, to castor oil can enhance its grounding effect. Rub your palms together, close your eyes, and take slow, deep breaths, focusing on the warmth and sensation of the oil. This simple ritual can become a soothing part of your morning or bedtime routine, creating a space for stillness in the midst of a busy day.

2. Emotional Release through Journaling and Self-Massage

Emotional wellness requires regular self-reflection and release. Holding onto emotions—whether it's stress, anger, or sadness—can lead to both physical and mental tension. Journaling is a powerful way to process emotions, but adding a castor oil self-massage afterward can provide physical relief that complements the emotional release.

To practice this, take 10-15 minutes each day to write freely about your thoughts and feelings. After journaling, apply a small amount of castor oil to areas where you feel physical tension, such as the neck, shoulders, or temples. Massaging these areas in circular motions while taking deep breaths can help release built-up stress and ease muscular tension, allowing both body and mind to relax.

3. Calming Breathwork and Castor Oil Application

Deep, intentional breathing is one of the most effective tools for calming the nervous system and promoting emotional balance. Breathwork practices, such as diaphragmatic breathing or the 4-7-8 breathing technique, can be enhanced by the comforting sensation of castor oil applied to pressure points.

To do this, apply a small amount of castor oil mixed with a drop or two of an essential oil like frankincense or ylang-ylang to pulse points on your wrists and neck. As you engage in your breathing practice, focus on the warmth of the oil on your skin. This combination of scent and sensation reinforces the calming effect of breathwork, helping you enter a state of deep relaxation. Use this technique before bed to ease into restful sleep or during moments of heightened stress to center yourself.

4. Using Castor Oil in Meditation for Emotional Balance

Meditation is a cornerstone of emotional wellness, allowing us to quiet the mind, observe our thoughts without judgment, and cultivate inner peace. Adding castor oil to your meditation routine can provide a tangible connection to the practice, deepening the sense of grounding and calm.

Before beginning your meditation, apply a small amount of castor oil to your hands and rub them together to generate warmth. Gently place your hands on your heart or abdomen and close your eyes. As you meditate, focus on the sensation of your hands and the warmth of the oil, helping you stay present in your body. The slow absorption of castor oil can make your meditation feel more immersive, connecting the physical and emotional aspects of relaxation. Over time, this practice can foster greater self-awareness, emotional resilience, and a sense of inner peace.

5. Creating an Evening Wind-Down Ritual with Castor Oil

An evening routine is essential for winding down from the day's activities and transitioning into a restful night's sleep. A calming evening ritual with castor oil can help your mind and body prepare for sleep, reducing the mental chatter and emotional residue that often lingers at the end of the day.

Begin by applying castor oil to your feet, massaging each toe and the soles of your feet. Feet are highly sensitive, with numerous pressure points that can affect the entire body. Massaging them with castor oil, particularly with added essential oils like cedarwood or chamomile, can help release stress and promote relaxation. This soothing ritual signals to your body that it's time to unwind, making it easier to fall asleep and wake up feeling refreshed.

CASTOR OIL FOR MENTAL CLARITY

Mental clarity is crucial for making decisions, staying focused, and managing our daily lives effectively. When we feel mentally clear, we're less prone to distractions, more productive, and better equipped to handle stress. Castor oil can be incorporated into routines that support mental clarity by enhancing focus and grounding practices. Used in combination with essential oils known for their cognitive benefits, castor oil can help reduce mental fog, promote alertness, and create a sense of mental freshness.

1. Morning Focus Ritual with Castor Oil and Essential Oils
Starting your day with a brief focus ritual can help set a productive tone for the hours ahead. A simple morning application of castor oil, paired with an invigorating essential oil like rosemary or peppermint, can sharpen your mental focus and wake up your senses.

Before you begin your day, apply a small amount of castor oil mixed with 2-3 drops of rosemary essential oil to your temples and neck. As you apply it, take a few moments to set your intentions for the day. Focus on inhaling the scent deeply, visualizing a day of clarity and productivity. This mindful ritual can help reduce morning fog and prepare you mentally for the tasks ahead.

2. Midday Rejuvenation with a Castor Oil Head Massage
During the day, mental fatigue can set in, making it difficult to concentrate. A quick head massage with castor oil can provide a refreshing mental break, helping you return to your tasks with renewed focus.

Warm a small amount of castor oil between your palms and gently massage it into your scalp, using circular motions. As you do so, visualize releasing any mental tension, clearing away distractions, and creating space for fresh ideas. This rejuvenating practice can be particularly beneficial during a lunch break or in the afternoon when focus tends to dip.

3. Enhancing Memory and Focus with Castor Oil and Essential Oils
Certain essential oils, such as basil and sage, are known for their cognitive benefits and can be paired with castor oil to create blends that support memory and concentration. This combination is ideal for students, professionals, or anyone who wants to enhance mental clarity and recall.

Mix a few drops of basil and sage essential oils with castor oil, and apply the blend to your temples, wrists, or neck before tasks that require focus, such as studying, working on a project, or preparing for a meeting. This practice not only promotes mental clarity but also enhances your ability to stay present and engaged with the task at hand.

4. Creating a Castor Oil Diffusion Space for Mental Clarity
Diffusing a blend of castor oil and essential oils in your workspace can create an environment that supports mental clarity. Although castor oil itself is too thick for diffusers, you can place a small bowl with castor oil mixed with essential oils on your desk to emit a subtle, refreshing scent throughout the day.

Add energizing essential oils like peppermint, eucalyptus, or lemon to castor oil and place it in an open dish or bowl near your workspace. As you work, the gentle aroma can help maintain mental clarity, reduce stress, and keep you alert.

This practice can be especially beneficial during long hours of focused work or study sessions.

5. Nightly Mental Decluttering with Castor Oil Application

Just as a morning focus ritual prepares you for the day, a nightly mental decluttering ritual can help you release the mental load accumulated throughout the day. This practice can improve your quality of sleep and allow you to wake up feeling refreshed.

Before bed, apply castor oil to your temples and neck, gently massaging these areas to release any lingering tension. As you do so, take a few deep breaths, focusing on each breath to quiet the mind. Imagine any stress or worry from the day melting away as you exhale. This nightly practice can help you clear mental clutter, allowing you to rest deeply and wake up ready for a new day.

INTEGRATING CASTOR OIL INTO YOUR EMOTIONAL AND MENTAL WELLNESS ROUTINE

Incorporating castor oil into your emotional and mental wellness routines doesn't have to be complicated. The practices described in this chapter offer simple yet powerful ways to enhance emotional balance and mental clarity. From grounding rituals to focus applications, each technique serves as a reminder to slow down, take a breath, and reconnect with your inner calm.

By building these rituals into your daily routine, you can create a foundation for emotional resilience and mental sharpness. Remember, wellness is a journey, and each small act of self-care brings you closer to a balanced, centered state of being. Whether you're just starting to explore natural wellness practices or looking to deepen your existing routine, castor oil is a gentle, effective ally in your pursuit of emotional balance and mental clarity.

Embrace these rituals with patience, allowing them to become moments of peace and intention in your daily life. As you cultivate emotional wellness and mental clarity, you may find yourself more capable of handling life's challenges, connecting deeply with others, and achieving a sense of fulfillment and harmony that enriches every aspect of your life.

APPENDIX 5
CASTOR OIL IN SPORTS AND FITNESS RECOVERY

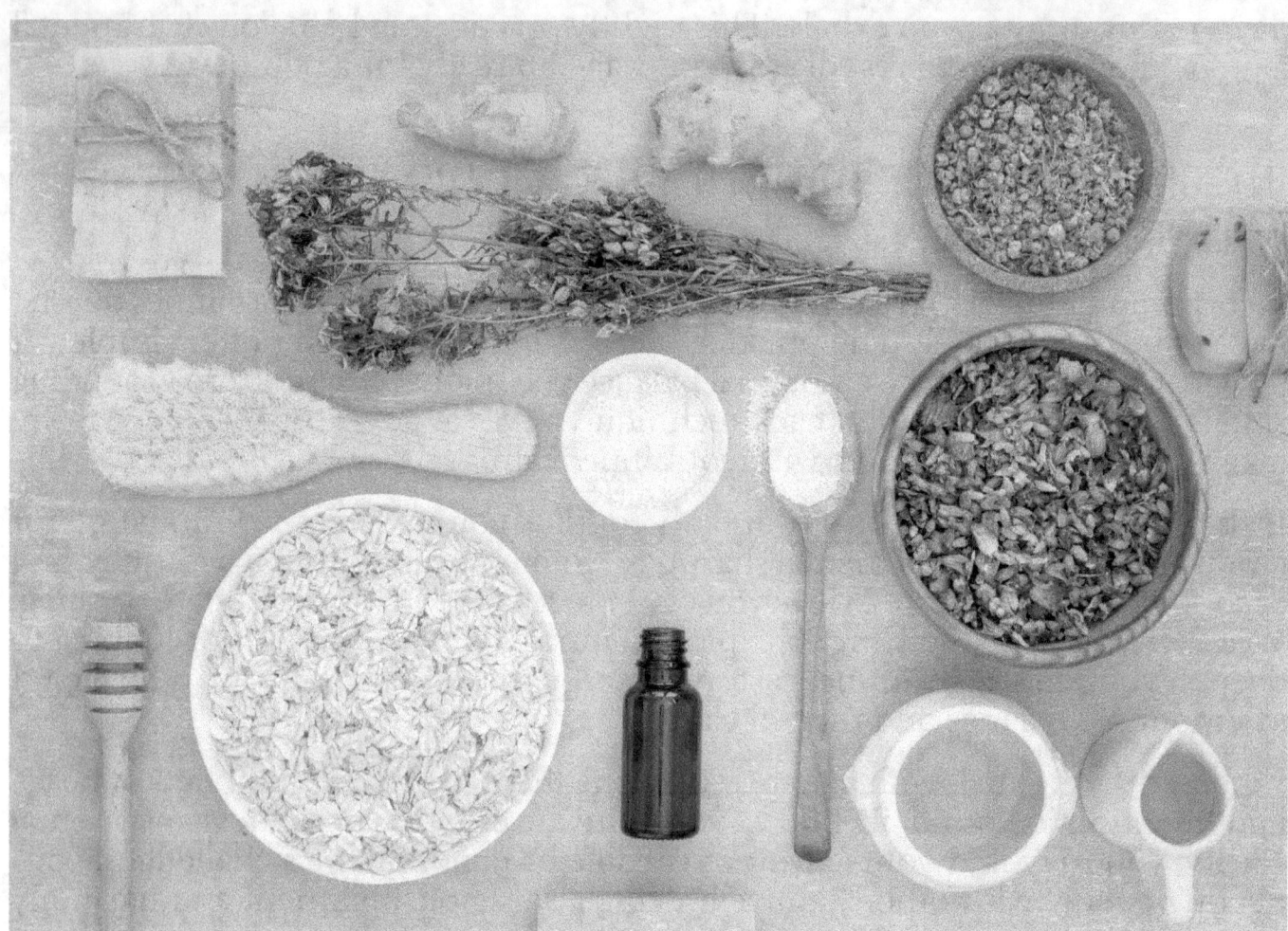

For athletes, fitness enthusiasts, and anyone engaged in regular physical activity, recovery is an essential part of maintaining peak performance and avoiding injuries. Recovery allows the body to repair itself, adapt, and grow stronger, setting the foundation for achieving fitness goals and sustaining a healthy, active lifestyle. Castor oil, known for its anti-inflammatory, pain-relieving, and skin-nourishing properties, can play an important role in sports and fitness recovery routines. This chapter delves into the benefits of castor oil for active individuals, with specific insights into how it supports muscle recovery, joint flexibility, and overall physical well-being.

BENEFITS OF CASTOR OIL FOR ACTIVE LIFESTYLES

For those who live an active lifestyle, regular exercise and physical activity can lead to muscle strain, soreness, joint stiffness, and even injuries. Managing these issues effectively is essential for consistent progress, longevity in sports, and overall physical health. Castor oil has several qualities that make it ideal for active people:

Anti-Inflammatory Properties: The ricinoleic acid in castor oil is a powerful anti-inflammatory agent, making it effective for reducing muscle soreness and joint inflammation. After intense workouts or physically demanding activities, inflammation naturally occurs as part of the body's repair process. However, excessive inflammation can cause prolonged soreness and discomfort. Castor oil's anti-inflammatory properties can help manage this inflammation, allowing muscles and joints to recover faster.

Pain Relief: Castor oil has natural analgesic (pain-relieving) qualities. When applied topically, it can provide relief from muscle aches and joint pain, making it useful for individuals who experience discomfort from rigorous physical activities. A gentle castor oil massage on sore areas can help reduce pain and improve comfort, whether you're recovering from an intense workout or managing chronic pain from sports-related injuries.

Moisturizing and Skin Protection: Physical activity, especially outdoor sports, can often lead to dry, chapped skin. Castor oil's moisturizing properties help keep the skin hydrated and protected from environmental damage caused by sun, wind, and other elements. Applying castor oil to the skin before and after physical activities can prevent dryness and irritation, helping you maintain healthy, resilient skin.

Deep Penetration for Muscle Relief: Unlike some topical oils, castor oil penetrates deeply into the skin and muscles, delivering its healing properties to the areas that need them most. This deep penetration allows it to provide relief for sore, tense muscles, making it an excellent addition to any recovery routine. It's particularly effective when used as a massage oil, as it softens and relaxes muscles while delivering nutrients and hydration.

Joint Flexibility Support: Castor oil's anti-inflammatory and moisturizing properties make it beneficial for joint health. By regularly applying castor oil to the knees, elbows, and other frequently used joints, you can help reduce stiffness and promote flexibility. Joint flexibility is crucial for injury prevention, as well as for maintaining performance and mobility over time.

Natural and Safe for Daily Use: Unlike many synthetic sports creams and ointments, castor oil is a natural, safe, and gentle option for daily use. It's free from harsh chemicals and additives, which makes it suitable for people with sensitive skin or those who prefer natural alternatives for their health and wellness needs.

CASTOR OIL FOR MUSCLE RECOVERY AND FLEXIBILITY

Muscle recovery is one of the most important aspects of physical training. Without adequate recovery, muscles don't have the chance to rebuild and grow, leading to fatigue, soreness, and even injury. Castor oil can be a valuable ally in the recovery process, providing deep muscle relief and flexibility support through various applications. Below are some specific ways castor oil can enhance muscle recovery and promote flexibility.

1. Pre-Workout Preparation with Castor Oil

Warming up before a workout is essential for reducing the risk of injury and improving performance. A pre-workout warm-up oil made with castor oil can help increase blood flow to the muscles, making them more pliable and ready for movement. Adding essential oils like rosemary or eucalyptus to castor oil can enhance its warming and circulation-boosting effects, ensuring muscles are well-prepared for physical exertion.

Apply the warm-up oil to major muscle groups, like the legs, arms, and back, before starting your warm-up exercises. This practice can help you enter your workout feeling more flexible, reducing the chances of strains or pulls.

2. Post-Workout Recovery and Soreness Relief

After a workout, it's common to experience soreness, especially if the session was particularly intense. A post-workout recovery balm made with castor oil can help reduce soreness and speed up recovery. This balm provides both anti-inflammatory and analgesic benefits, making it ideal for soothing overworked muscles.

Massaging castor oil onto sore areas can help promote circulation, which aids in removing lactic acid buildup—a common cause of post-exercise soreness. The massage also stimulates lymphatic drainage, helping your body eliminate toxins and waste products produced during intense physical activity.

3. Enhancing Joint Flexibility with Castor Oil Packs

Joint flexibility is crucial for athletes and active individuals, as it reduces the likelihood of injuries and improves performance. Castor oil packs are a great way to deliver deep relief to stiff joints, promoting flexibility and mobility over time. By placing a warm castor oil pack on the knees, elbows, shoulders, or any other joints, you can help relax the muscles and tendons surrounding the joint, making it easier to move and stretch.

To create a castor oil pack, soak a cloth in castor oil and apply it to the affected area, covering it with a heating pad. This method allows the oil to penetrate deeply, delivering its anti-inflammatory and pain-relieving properties directly to the joint.

4. Muscle Relaxation and Recovery through Castor Oil Baths

A warm bath infused with castor oil can be an incredibly relaxing and effective way to promote muscle recovery. The heat from the bath helps muscles relax, while the castor oil's soothing properties provide additional relief for sore or tense areas. Adding Epsom salts and essential oils to the bath can further enhance relaxation and support muscle healing.

After an intense workout or a long day of physical activity, a castor oil bath can serve as a restorative practice, helping you unwind and rejuvenate.

5. Tendon and Ligament Support with Castor Oil

Tendons and ligaments are highly susceptible to strain during intense physical activities. Applying castor oil to these areas can help reduce inflammation and support healing, especially when combined with essential oils like frankincense or helichrysum, known for their joint-supporting properties.

Castor oil massages on the ankles, wrists, and knees can help strengthen the tendons and ligaments over time, improving stability and reducing the likelihood of strains and sprains.

REMEDIES FOR SPORTS AND FITNESS RECOVERY

Below are some specific remedies that utilize castor oil to support sports and fitness recovery. These remedies are easy to prepare and can become valuable additions to any fitness routine.

1. Pre-Workout Muscle Warm-Up Oil

Purpose: Increases blood flow to muscles, making them more pliable and prepared for exercise.

INGREDIENTS

- 2 tablespoons castor oil
- 5 drops rosemary essential oil (for circulation)
- 3 drops eucalyptus essential oil (for warming effect)

INSTRUCTIONS

1. In a small bottle, combine the castor oil with the essential oils.
2. Shake well to blend.

How to Use: Apply the warm-up oil to major muscle groups before warming up. Massage gently to increase blood flow and warm the muscles.

2. Post-Workout Soreness Relief Balm

Purpose: Reduces muscle soreness and aids recovery after intense exercise.

INGREDIENTS

- 2 tablespoons castor oil
- 1 tablespoon shea butter (optional, for extra moisture)
- 5 drops lavender essential oil (for relaxation)
- 5 drops peppermint essential oil (for cooling)

INSTRUCTIONS

1. Melt the shea butter and mix it with castor oil.
2. Add the essential oils and stir well.
3. Pour into a small container and let it set.

How to Use: Apply to sore muscles after a workout to reduce pain and promote relaxation.

3. Joint Flexibility Castor Oil Pack

Purpose: Provides deep relief to stiff joints, enhancing flexibility and mobility.

INGREDIENTS

- 1/4 cup castor oil
- A soft cloth or cotton flannel
- Heating pad

INSTRUCTIONS

1. Soak the cloth in castor oil and apply it to the affected joint.
2. Place a heating pad over the cloth and let it sit for 20-30 minutes.

How to Use: Use on joints like knees, elbows, or shoulders to relieve stiffness and support flexibility.

4. Muscle Relaxation Bath Soak

Purpose: Helps relax muscles and reduces soreness after intense physical activity.

INGREDIENTS

- 2 tablespoons castor oil
- 1 cup Epsom salts (for magnesium and muscle relief)
- 5 drops lavender essential oil (for relaxation)
- 3 drops chamomile essential oil (for soothing)

INSTRUCTIONS

1. Combine the Epsom salts and essential oils.
2. Add the mixture to a warm bath, and drizzle in castor oil.

How to Use: Soak in the bath for 20-30 minutes after a workout or physically demanding day.

5. Tendon and Ligament Support Balm

Purpose: Supports tendons and ligaments, reducing inflammation and strengthening these crucial structures.

INGREDIENTS

- 2 tablespoons castor oil
- 5 drops frankincense essential oil (for joint support)
- 3 drops helichrysum essential oil (for healing properties)

INSTRUCTIONS

1. In a small bottle, combine castor oil with the essential oils.
2. Shake well to blend.

How to Use: Apply to the ankles, wrists, and knees to support tendons and ligaments after exercise.

INTEGRATING CASTOR OIL INTO A SPORTS AND FITNESS RECOVERY ROUTINE

The above remedies demonstrate the versatility of castor oil as a natural and effective tool for fitness recovery. By adding these practices into your regular routine, you can support muscle recovery, improve joint flexibility, and reduce the discomfort associated with intense physical activity. Castor oil's anti-inflammatory, pain-relieving, and moisturizing properties make it particularly valuable for those who lead active lives.

Remember, consistency is key to seeing the best results. By making castor oil a regular part of your sports and fitness recovery, you're not only taking care of your body but also enhancing your performance and resilience. Embrace the power of natural recovery, and let castor oil support you in achieving your fitness goals with health, comfort, and longevity in mind.

CONCLUSION

Congratulations on reaching the end of this journey into the transformative world of castor oil! From ancient practices to modern applications, castor oil stands out as a remarkably versatile tool, offering solutions for health, beauty, and overall well-being. As you've discovered, castor oil isn't just a remedy from the past; it's a gift of nature that continues to support us in countless ways, promoting holistic health with simplicity and effectiveness.

Throughout this exploration, we've seen castor oil's potential to enhance our lives with gentle care, whether through skin rejuvenation, pain relief, digestive support, or non-toxic cleaning solutions. Each recipe and remedy shared is an invitation to step into a more natural, intentional lifestyle, reminding us of the powerful alternatives that exist beyond synthetic products. What's wonderful about castor oil is its accessibility and ease—there's no complicated process or hefty cost involved. A single bottle of castor oil opens doors to an array of benefits that fit seamlessly into your daily routine.

As you've read, castor oil allows for easy integration into your life. There's no need to overhaul your entire wellness approach at once. Begin with small steps, perhaps by adding castor oil to your nightly routine to relax your muscles or soothe your skin. Little by little, you'll discover how simple it is to incorporate these natural remedies into your life in a way that feels both rewarding and manageable. Soon enough, castor oil becomes a comforting part of your routine, supporting you in times of stress, nourishing your body, and adding moments of mindful care to your day.

One of the most inspiring aspects of working with natural remedies like castor oil is the opportunity to create your own solutions tailored to your personal needs. There's something incredibly empowering about mixing up your own face serum, massage oil, or cleaning spray. These aren't just products; they're small acts of self-care and connection to nature, crafted with your own hands and intentions. In a world that often pushes us to buy more, faster, or "better," castor oil offers a refreshingly simple reminder of the value of creating and personalizing what we use.

Natural wellness is an ever-evolving journey, one that grows and shifts with each new discovery. Castor oil is just one of many resources available to you, but it's a gateway to understanding and embracing the healing power of simplicity. By working with castor oil, you might feel inspired to learn more about other oils, herbs, or natural wellness practices that resonate with you. Each new experience and experiment builds confidence and trust in your ability to care for yourself in ways that align with your values and needs.

As you deepen your understanding of castor oil's benefits, remember that these remedies are gifts meant to be shared. If you have friends or family curious about natural wellness, why not teach them a few of the remedies you've tried? Show them how easy it is to make a castor oil hand cream or a soothing massage balm. Sharing the knowledge you've gained creates a ripple effect, encouraging others to explore natural solutions and discover the joys of simple, intentional living. Imagine a world where wellness is built on community knowledge, where we empower each other to find natural solutions that work for our unique needs.

You may even find yourself passing these recipes down through generations, creating a legacy of health and care. Introducing castor oil into your family's routine can teach children about the importance of nature and self-care. This knowledge becomes a valuable tool they can carry with them, helping them make mindful choices about their own wellness in the future.

Looking ahead, castor oil offers the flexibility to adapt to your evolving needs. Whether you're addressing skin changes, sore muscles, or seasonal health shifts, castor oil remains a constant, supporting you through different stages and moments of life. As you continue this journey, feel free to revisit the recipes and adapt them as you grow. Wellness is a lifelong practice, and the routines you create now can be enjoyed for years to come, shaping a lifestyle that nurtures your mind, body, and spirit.

Choosing to incorporate natural remedies like castor oil into your life is a meaningful step toward a balanced, sustainable way of living. It's an investment not just in your health but in the values you hold—respect for your body, for nature, and for simplicity. Each time you reach for your bottle of castor oil, you're choosing a path that celebrates slow, intentional wellness over quick fixes. These choices add up, creating a lifestyle that feels aligned, purposeful, and empowering.

This journey into the world of castor oil has been about more than learning recipes; it's been about reconnecting with the wisdom of nature and rediscovering our own power to heal, nurture, and support ourselves. There's a special kind of satisfaction that comes from knowing you can make small, effective changes in your life with just a few simple ingredients. This journey is about embracing that feeling, about valuing progress over perfection, and about creating a wellness practice that grows with you, one that feels personal and enriching.

Thank you for diving into this exploration of castor oil with curiosity and openness. May your journey with this natural remedy continue to bring you comfort, health, and joy. As you close this book, I hope you feel inspired, equipped, and ready to make castor oil a meaningful part of your wellness routine. Here's to a future filled with discovery, balance, and the simple beauty of natural health.

Enjoy every moment of this journey, knowing that with each new use of castor oil, you're choosing wellness, simplicity, and a deep respect for the gifts of nature.

YOUR EXCLUSIVE BONUS

10 Hours of video on Castor Oil

INDEX

A

Acne Scar Healing Mask 27
Aftershave Moisturizing Lotion 73
All-Purpose Household Cleaner 79
Aloe and Castor After-Sun Lotion 110
Anti-Aging Castor Oil Night Cream 26
Anti-Anxiety Body Balm 95
Anti-Cramping Salve 60
Anti-Dandruff Scalp Treatment 34
Anti-Frizz Hair Serum 35
Anti-Fungal Paw Spray 89
Anti-Itch Remedy for Pets 86
Arthritis Relief Rub 42
Athlete's Foot Relief Balm 75

B

Baby Massage Oil 67
Bathroom Scrub with Castor Oil 81
Beard Growth Serum 75
Beard Oil Blend 71
Bloating Reduction Tincture 50
Breast Health Castor Oil Pack 59
Bug Bite Soother 65
Burn Relief Ointment 21

C

Calming Chest Rub 113
Calming Massage Oil 93
Carpet Stain Remover 82
Castor Oil and Calendula Healing Salve 108
Castor Oil and Ginger Tea 53
Castor Oil and Turmeric Brightening Mask 27
Castor Oil Aromatherapy Blend 93
Castor Oil-Based Deodorant 112
Castor Oil Compress for Soreness 22
Castor Oil Detox Drink 49
Castor Oil Ear Mite Treatment 90
Castor Oil Eye Serum 21
Castor Oil Face Glow Serum 29
Castor Oil Face Scrub 76
Castor Oil Foot Scrub 109
Castor Oil for Pet Skin Allergies 90
Castor Oil for Pet Wounds 89
Castor Oil Furniture Polish 79
Castor Oil Hair Detangler 114
Castor Oil Hair Sealant 38
Castor Oil Hair Thickening Gel 76
Castor Oil Head Massage for Relaxation 95
Castor Oil Healing Salve 19
Castor Oil Heat Pack for Back Pain 43
Castor Oil Infused Herbal Tincture 106
Castor Oil Knee Wrap 45
Castor Oil Lavender Eye Compress 94
Castor Oil Makeup Remover 28
Castor Oil Meditation Balm 95
Castor Oil Mold and Mildew Remover 81
Castor Oil Overnight Hair Treatment 37
Castor Oil Pack for Sore Muscles 42
Castor Oil Pain Relief Pack 41
Castor Oil Relaxation Candle 97
Castor Oil Roll-On Pain Reliever 107
Castor Oil Room Spray 83
Castor Oil Rub for Joint Flexibility 74
Castor Oil Solid Perfume 111
Castor Oil Split-End Mender 35
Castor Oil Stretch Mark Cream 115
Castor Oil Tincture for Immune Health 115
Chakra Aligning Oil Blend 101
Children's Immune Boost Balm 67
Children's Tummy Relief Pack 65
Circulation-Boosting Foot Rub 74
Circulation Enhancing Balm 103
Cleansing Oil for Face 113
Coat Shine Serum 90
Cold Relief Chest Compress 68
Colic Relief Massage Oil 64
Colon Cleanse Castor Oil Drink 51
Color Protection Hair Serum 36
Constipation Relief Remedy 50
Cooling Relief Gel 114
Cuticle Oil for Nail Health 108

D

Dark Spot Correcting Serum 27
Deep Conditioning Castor Oil Hair Mask 34
Deep Moisturizing Hand Cream 109
Deep Pore Cleansing Oil 29
Deep Tissue Relief Oil 101
Detoxifying Foot Balm 102
Digestive Enzyme Support 52
Digestive Support Tonic 50
DIY Anti-Itch Spray 107
DIY Candle with Castor Oil 97

DIY Hand Sanitizer with Castor Oil 110
DIY Makeup Remover Wipes 113
DIY Perfume Balm with Castor Oil 109
DIY Sleep Aid Balm 94
Dry Scalp Hydration Serum 35

E

Earache Relief Pack 68
Ear Cleaning Solution 87
Elbow and Wrist Relief Balm 45
Energy Balancing Body Balm 100
Energy Boost Massage Oil 74

F

Fertility Enhancing Castor Pack 58
Fine Line Smoothing Cream 28
Flea Prevention Rub 87
Foot Hydrating Mask 114
Foot Pain Relief Balm 44
Foot Soak for Stress Relief 94

G

Gallbladder Support Pack 53
Gentle Chest Rub for Colds 64
Gentle Eczema Balm 66
Gentle Laxative Blend 51
Gut Health Smoothie 49

H

Hair and Scalp Strengthening Oil 72
Hair Growth Oil Blend 34
Hair Shine Serum 112
Hair Strengthening Serum 37
Hand and Nail Moisturizing Treatment 97
Hand Hydration Cream 23
Healing Balm for Paws and Skin 86
Herbal Healing Oil for Skin Rejuvenation 116
Herbal Infusion Oil 111
Hormone-Balancing Body Lotion 57
Hot Flash Relief Balm 59
Hot Oil Treatment for Scalp 38
Hot Spot Relief Gel 88
Hydrating Face Mist 30

I

Immune-Boosting Castor Oil 101
Inflammation-Reducing Massage Oil 41
Insect Repellent Balm 111
Intestinal Healing Tea 52

J

Joint and Muscle Pain Salve 42
Joint Flexibility Castor Oil Pack 126

K

Kitchen Degreaser 83

L

Laundry Stain Remover 80
Leave-In Conditioner with Castor Oil 36
Libido Support Massage Oil 59
Lip Repair Balm 21
Liver Detox Castor Pack 51

M

Menopause Support Cream 58
Menstrual Pain Relief Castor Oil Pack 57
Migraine Relief Castor Compress 44
Mild Castor Oil Salve for Cuts 65
Mild Sunburn Relief Gel 68
Mind-Body Wellness Oil 100
Moisturizing Body Balm 20
Mood-Boosting Roller Blend 96
Muscle Recovery Rub 73
Muscle Relaxation Bath Soak 126

N

Natural Anti-Tick Oil 88
Natural Beard Softener 72
Natural Bug Bite Soother 115
Natural Castor Oil Soap 79
Natural Dish Soap 80
Natural Laxative Capsules 53
Natural Lip Balm with Castor Oil 108
Natural Sunscreen with Castor Oil 106
Nerve Pain Relief Oil 43

O

Oil-Free Moisturizer 31
Ovarian Support Tincture 60
Oven and Grill Cleaner 82

P

Paw Pad Protector 87
PCOS Support Serum 61
Peaceful Sleep Pillow Spray 96
Perimenopause Symptom Relief Oil 60
Pet Odor Remover 89
Pet Relaxation Massage Oil 88
Pet-Safe Floor Cleaner 80
Pet Shampoo 86
Pigmentation Reduction Oil 31
PMS Relief Massage Oil 58
Post-Exercise Recovery Balm 102
Post-Shave Skin Balm 72
Post-Workout Soreness Relief Balm 126
Prenatal Skin Support Balm 61
Pre-Workout Muscle Warm-Up Oil 125
Pre-Workout Warm-Up Oil 75

Prostate Health Castor Pack 73

R

Rash and Itch Relief Lotion 67
Reflexology Massage Oil 102
Relaxing Bath Soak with Castor Oil and Essential Oils 93
Relaxing Massage Balm 112
Reproductive Health Tea 61
Ricinoleic Acid Skin Serum 19

S

Scalp Exfoliating Treatment 36
Scalp Soothing Spray 37
Scar Healing Solution 20
Sciatica Pain Relief Pack 44
Silver Polish 83
Skin Detoxifying Mask 30
Skin Firming Lotion 28
Sleep Support Castor Pack 103
Sleep Support Oil Blend 66
Smoothing Body Butter 110
Soothing Diaper Rash Balm 64
Soothing Moisturizing Lotion 106
Soothing Skin Balm 22
Sore Neck Relief Oil 45
Stomach Gas Relief Pack 53
Stomach Soothing Castor Oil Rub 52
Stress-Reducing Body Oil 96
Stretch Mark Healing Oil 57

T

Teething Relief Rub 66
Tendon and Ligament Support Balm 127
Tendonitis Support Balm 43
Tension Headache Balm 45
Thinning Hair Support Oil 38
Toilet Bowl Cleaner 82

U

Under Eye Dark Circle Balm 30

V

Vitamin E Infused Body Oil 107

W

Window and Glass Cleaner 81
Wrinkle-Reducing Eye Cream 29

www.ingramcontent.com/pod-product-compliance
Lightning Source LLC
Chambersburg PA
CBHW080458220526
45465CB00006B/2312